Five Simple Steps

TO

Emotional Healing

THE LAST
SELF-HELP
BOOK YOU
WILL EVER
NEED

Gloria Arenson, MS, MFT

A FIRESIDE BOOK
PUBLISHED BY SIMON & SCHUSTER
NEW YORK LONDON TORONTO SYDNEY SINGAPORE

Note/Caveat

The information and suggestions contained in this book are not intended as a substitute for appropriate medical or mental health treatment. Please consult your health practitioner when you are dealing with serious problems.

The stories contained in this book are often composites created from the many clients I have treated over the years.

FIRESIDE
Rockefeller Center
1230 Avenue of the Americas
New York, NY 10020

FIRESIDE and colophon are registered
trademarks of Simon & Schuster, Inc.

Designed by Christine Weathersbee

Manufactured in the United States of America

10 9 8 7 6 5 4 3 2 1

Library of Congress Cataloging-in-Publication Data
Arenson, Gloria

Five simple steps to emotional healing : the last self-help book you will
ever need / Gloria Arenson.
p. cm.
Includes bibliographical references and index.
1. Acupuncture points. 2. Acupuncture. I. Title.
RM184.5 .A745 2001
618.8'92—dc21   2001040677
ISBN 0-7432-1387-4

Dedication

This book is dedicated to everyone who reads it. My dream is to teach the world to use Meridian Therapy. I envision a world in which teachers employ this technique to help their students learn better and cooperate more, and to give children a tool they can use throughout their lives. I envision doctors, dentists, and nurses using Meridian Therapy to help their patients cope with pain and fear. I envision a world in which families tap together and spouses use Meridian Therapy to resolve anger and frustration so they can communicate more clearly.

Imagine a world where people take a few minutes each day to eliminate anger, fear, worry, pain, and grief. I think we will see less violence and more love. Peace on earth can start at your fingertips.

Share this book with your children, parents, spouses, lovers, friends, and coworkers. Spread the word.

Acknowledgments

I thank Gary Craig for leading the way into a new world of healing possibility. His creativity, inspiration, and generosity changed my life personally and professionally. Gary's willingness to support all of us who want to help build the "healing high-rise" is awe-inspiring.

I appreciate all my Meridian Therapy colleagues on the Internet around the world who have questioned, shared information and cases, and always treated each other with love and respect. Thank you to Fred Gallo, Willem Lammers, Don Elium, and David Grudermeyer for keeping the lines of communication open.

Thanks to Terri Cooper, who told me that I would write this book before I ever thought of it. The assistance and feedback from Cynthia Anderson and Kathy Hardin was invaluable. I couldn't have asked for a better guide than my agent, Toni Lopopolo. I am grateful to my clients and friends who allowed me to share their intimate stories and triumphs. I am fortunate that my children, Leslie and Drew, were willing to tap along with me.

I could not have written this book without the love, support, and talent of my wonderful husband, Laurence Brockway.

CONTENTS

INTRODUCTION:
Join the Healing Revolution

I have been a licensed psychotherapist for more than twenty years, and I must begin my book with an apology to my readers. I apologize for being part of a group that has preached that you have to work long and hard in order to overcome emotional pain and suffering. Some of us have convinced you that the more pain you feel as you "work things through," the better the healing. You now believe that without pain you aren't making headway.

I want to assure you that we meant well. We didn't know any better. We worked with the tools at our disposal. And those tools were often primitive.

In the last ten years great strides have been made in the field of psychotherapy. Today, new *Power Therapies* are available that are generating innovative emotional healing techniques. These approaches are based on the awareness that we are a body/mind. Meridian Therapy is one of these.

Meridian Therapy is a procedure based on stimulating the energy meridians in the body by tapping on specific energy points. You can learn it in minutes and use it to eliminate a lifetime of fear, anxiety, grief, guilt, shame, cravings, traumatic memories, and more. Meridian Therapy works much faster than previous psychotherapies and accomplishes more without causing pain.

"But," you may exclaim, "I have to really understand what created this problem. I have to take time to talk about it." The most popular psychotherapeutic technique is "talk therapy." Many of you have talked and talked for years in order to understand yourself better, thinking that insights might make all the difference.

When I first went to a psychotherapist for talk therapy, many years ago, I often left the session in great emotional pain. We would open up subjects that were difficult to face, and when the hour was up, I had to leave, no matter where we were. Sometimes I could barely see as I drove home, because of the tears pouring from my eyes. "How am I going to get through the week until my next appointment?" I often asked myself.

I discovered that if I kept thinking about what was bothering me, and imagined what my therapist would say, I frequently resolved the issue without her help. The answer was always within me. I just had to learn how to retrieve it. Meridian Therapy is a technique that allows you do the same thing, only more efficiently and with less effort. You don't have to be in therapy to help yourself, using the suggestions in this book.

I used to tell my clients that talk therapy is like going fishing. We sat in the room together, like fishermen in a boat on a lake. We knew that there were fish in there, but we couldn't see them. The fish we sought were healing moments. We spent the time casting our lines into the waters of the mind. Sometimes we got a nibble but came up empty. Other times, we caught a big one. We won some, we lost some. We kept trying, week in and week out.

With Meridian Therapy you don't have to fish around. You go directly to the healing power within you. You will rarely come up empty. Each time you use this technique, healing takes place. The process is so streamlined that it takes much less time to work through problems than using traditional "talk therapy" or other self-help approaches. And, best of all, you can use it by yourself on most of life's problems.

Power Therapies such as NLP (Neuro Linguistic Programming), EMDR (Eye Movement Desensitization and Reprocessing), and TFT (Thought Field Therapy) are now in the public domain. These healing methods, compared to those you may have experienced in the past, are like lasers as compared to an old hammer. They help you target the problem more efficiently and heal deeply and permanently.

Ever since Roger Callahan developed Thought Field Therapy, the first tapping technique that can heal in minutes, his followers have worked to refine and improve this process. Each one has given his variation a special name. Gary Craig formulated Emotional Freedom Techniques, James V. Durlacher practices Acu-POWER, and Larry Nims teaches Be Set Free Fast. Fred Gallo and Greg Nicosia have also created wonderful energy meridian techniques.

Meridian Therapy is the name I have used to encompass all these tapping techniques. We are only at the beginning of a powerful new way of treating emotional problems. Meridian Therapy synthesizes the best aspects of all these tapping techniques into a single, easy-to-use system.

In this book:
- I will tell you about the scientific basis of Meridian Therapy.
- I will show you how to practice it on yourself.

- I will give you detailed instructions for applying Meridian Therapy in many areas of your life.

You will learn how to:
- Dissolve negative emotions, anger, sadness, fear, guilt, and shame.
- Eliminate panic attacks and phobias.
- Solve problems in your daily life immediately.
- Overcome procrastination and addictive cravings.
- Improve your performance in sports, work, and even sex.
- Enhance physical well-being and relieve pain.

You can learn how to practice Meridian Therapy in minutes and use it anywhere, any time. Wherever you are, it is as close as your fingertips.

Deepak Chopra has said there is a difference between pain and suffering. Pain is necessary for your health because it tells you that something is wrong, especially in the medical sense. Suffering, however, is self-inflicted. If you are ready to give up your suffering, read on.

Part One

Your Meridian Therapy Tool Kit

chapter one

Meridian Therapy: What It's All About

Meridian Therapy is a self-healing approach based on the view that the body and mind are inextricably intertwined, and healing happens in both areas. We must trust that the body/mind we call our "self" has innate wisdom and will provide whatever each of us needs in order to restore health. Meridian Therapy is a powerful technique that encourages any emotional healing that needs to take place. Healing occurs when we tune in to the problem while gently tapping acupuncture points on the face, hands, and upper body to balance the energy.

How It Works

The goal of Meridian Therapy is to heal emotional problems. The theory behind this technique is that old emotional wounds are stored in the body as blocked energetic patterns.

Stimulating energy points removes the disturbance, allowing our body/mind system to process the troubling problem. As the energy is brought into balance, worrisome thoughts and memories about upsetting circumstances change and negative emotions diminish. This process takes place on a bioelectromagnetic level throughout our being.

The Mind in the Body

Where are feelings located? Are they in the brain? Most of us think that feelings originate in the brain, but the renowned neurobiologist Candace Pert, Ph.D., has discovered that emotions are in the body as well as in the brain. In her research she proved that there are emotional receptors in cells throughout the body. The "unconscious" is not in the brain, she says, but is present everywhere in the whole system of the body. She calls this the Bodymind. According to her findings there is constant intercellular communication between the brain, glands, and immune system.

East Meets West

In Meridian Therapy, modern-day psychology meets the ancient wisdom of the East to achieve healing. Almost five thousand years ago the Chinese knew that there was an energy component in the acupuncture meridians in the body. The twenty-four-volume *Nei Ching*, said to have been written by Huang Ti, the "Yellow Emperor," is the oldest known text about acupuncture and dates from about 2600 B.C. It describes the energy pathways we now call meridians and details acupuncture points.

The Chinese were not the only ancients to have this understanding of the bioelectromagnetic system of the body. The vital energy the Chinese call Chi was already known in India as Prana. In Egypt a papyrus dated 1150 B.C. describes something similar to meridians. Long ago, healers in Arabia and Brazil knew about the energy properties of the body, as did the Eskimos. In fact, every indigenous culture on earth has a term for this Vital Force: Wakan, Ki, Mana, and so forth.

While the meridians carry energy throughout the body, there are seven energy centers in the body called chakras. The concept of chakras was first developed in ancient India. Chakras act like transformers and convert subtle energies into chemical, hormonal, and cellular changes in the body. Candace Pert's research revealed that there are clusters of emotional receptor cells in the chakra areas.

Measuring the Vital Force

Instruments have measured the Chi or bioenergy flowing from the hands of modern chi-gong masters who are able to focus Chi energy and use it to heal. These people have learned how to harness the energy and direct it. We all have this same energy and can learn to use it. Every one of us has extremely low frequency energy radiating from different parts of our body. Our hands and forehead radiate the strongest energy.

Scientists have measured the intensity of these biophotons or light emissions. According to Beverly Rubik, Ph.D., a leading biophysicist and research pioneer; in recent experiments, meditation increased biophoton emissions from the crown of the head and the hands by factors of 100 to 1,000. Just thinking with intention about the Vital Force also increased the energy by the same factor. Living creatures both radiate and attract subtle energy. Dr. Rubik proposes that this subtle energy that we receive and emit may turn out to be even more fundamental than our biochemistry.

More About Meridian Pathways

"Meridians carry energy the way arteries carry blood," says Donna Eden, author of *Energy Medicine*. She describes the energy meridians as "the body's energy bloodstream." These meridians are dotted with hundreds of acupuncture points. Energy points are sensitive to bioelectric impulses in the body.

They are like antennae that transmit heat, electromagnetic energy, or the Vital Force (Chi). The meridians, deep inside the body, run through our organs and muscle groups like roadways that go from the top of the head to the tips of the toes. This energy communication system connects the organs and sensory and emotional aspects of the body. Thoughts have power, and negative thoughts can adversely affect the subtle energies carried by the meridians. Intense emotions can disrupt the energy flow as well.

Sometimes the meridian highways become backed up with too much energy and a bottleneck occurs. Our bodies operate twenty-four hours a day, seven days a week. Inevitably we experience stress. The energy pathways need to be kept free because disturbances can lead to ill health and emotional problems. Tapping specific acupuncture points gets the energy flowing smoothly and dissolves negative states. When free flow is restored, the negative emotional charge is eliminated and problems seem to melt away.

The ancient Chinese believed that emotions are concentrated in the meridians. They taught that pain and negative feelings such as anger, fear, guilt, confusion, and obsession lead to imbalance in the body's harmony. Emotional dysfunction indicates that there is a disturbance in the energy system. When that occurs, acupuncturists insert fine needles into specific points to balance the flow of energy. Acupressure is another healing method of pressing energy points on the skin to stimulate meridians rather than inserting needles. Both techniques move blocked energies and release many symptoms of illness or emotional problems.

Western Science Steps In

Although the Chinese have used acupuncture successfully for thousands of years, they could not prove their claims. Western society discounted this approach to healing until relatively recently. Independent of the culture of Asia, scientists since the eighteenth century have investigated the electromagnetic properties of life and discovered that complex energy fields surround every living thing. The flow of energy in the body has been traced along the same consistent pathways the Chinese know as energy meridians. With new technology it is now possible to measure that energy.

Most of us think of matter as one thing and energy as something else, but Albert Einstein demonstrated that matter and energy are interchangeable aspects of the same reality. Therefore, everything can be seen as a form of energy. We can think of ourselves as consisting not only of solid packets of energy (our bodies) but also of intangible packets of energy (our thoughts). Meridian Therapy helps rebalance our physical and mental energies, thereby optimizing our bioelectromagnetic state.

Fields of Life

Harold Saxton Burr, Ph.D., who taught anatomy and neuroanatomy at Yale University, measured electrical currents in and around life forms. He studied all kinds of living things from simple molds, worms, and trees to complex life systems such as human beings. He affirmed that we have "fields of life" or "L-fields," which are electromagnetic fields. These fields help stabilize the pattern each form takes so that all trees, animals, people, and so forth maintain the same shape and properties.

Proof That Energy Points Exist

Another pioneer in this work, Reinhold Voll, M.D., discovered that acupuncture points show a dramatic decrease in electrical resistance on the skin compared to nonacupuncture points. He and his associates also found that each point seemed to have a standard measurement for healthy individuals, but the measurements change when health deteriorates.

Drs. Robert O. Becker and Maria Reichmanis developed an electrode device that can be rolled along the meridians to measure electrical skin resistance and give a continuous reading. Their work confirmed that meridians have electrical qualities like transmission lines, and concluded that the acupuncture system was measurable.

In 1992 a study was conducted in France to prove that meridians exist. Over three hundred people took part. A radioactive tracer was injected at acupuncture points, and a special camera was able to image the path. A similar tracer was also injected at a control point that was not an acupuncture point. The tracer injected in the acupuncture points followed the same pathways described as meridians in traditional Chinese medicine. However, the tracer injected in the random points diffused. Each experiment was repeated several times.

Describing Subtle Energies

Stanford professor William A. Tiller, Ph.D., studies the "supersensible" domains of Nature—aspects of light, sound, space, and time that are beyond what we can sense. "Subtle energies are all those beyond the familiar ones associated with the four fundamental forces accepted by the conventional physics model," he says.

Dr. Tiller thinks of the whole body as an antenna with the potential to transmit and receive Chi energy. He surmises that when we touch an acupuncture point, we stimulate ion flow that reacts at the subtle energy level to unclog meridian channels. Applying this knowledge to the field of psychology brings about a dramatic shift in how emotional healing can take place. Extremely tiny energy signals can affect us and stimulate healing responses by coaxing the system back into normalcy.

Ancient Indian and Chinese healers understood the subtle energies before findings in the field of quantum physics helped us understand the nature of energy and matter. We now know that information carried by subtle energies can travel faster than the speed of light and that focusing thought energy can have an effect on matter.

Dr. Beverly Rubik hypothesizes that all living systems are permeated by an energy information flow. It is not the energy that heals, but rather the "intelligent" information transmitted bioenergetically. The energy signal carries the bioinformation necessary for healing. It is intangible, but cells can read the information that is delivered this way and respond. Recent experiments indicate that when love or unconditional acceptance are present the healings that result are even more impressive.

The Evolution of Meridian Therapy

Fred Gallo, Ph.D., in his book *Energy Psychology*, writes that thoughts exist in fields and negative emotions are rooted in energy configurations. "If thought and psychological problems exist in energy field form, then psychological problems can be resolved much more easily than one might assume. Based on the new paradigms, it would then be merely a matter of altering the energy field."

Meridian Therapy evolved from connecting these ideas about the energy systems of the body with a type of muscle testing frequently practiced by chiropractors. In muscle testing the individual is usually asked to hold out an arm and resist when the practitioner pushes firmly on the forearm. The arm will remain firm and strong when there is a positive thought or the answer is yes. When there is a negative thought or the answer is no, the arm will wobble. In the 1960s Dr. George Goodheart, a chiropractor, discovered a new way to diagnose his patients by testing the relative strength or weakness of muscles. This method is called Applied Kinesiology.

As he practiced this technique, Goodheart realized that there is a relationship between the muscles and other organs and glands in the body. When a particular muscle tested weak, a corresponding part of the body, such as the spleen, liver, or stomach, was found, through medical tests, to be dysfunctional. When Goodheart learned of the relationship between the muscles and meridian pathways, he began to use acupuncture in his practice. In addition to treating structural problems of the body, Applied Kinesiology treats mental conditions as well.

Behavioral Kinesiology

Psychiatrist John Diamond, M.D., believes that the body doesn't lie. In the 1970s, Diamond created Behavioral Kinesiology by incorporating Applied Kinesiology and psychotherapy. His method brings together ideas from psychiatry, psychosomatic medicine, music, and the humanities. Diamond asserts that an imbalance of Chi, or Vital Force, affects a specific energy meridian and leads to psychological and physical problems.

Using muscle testing, Diamond connected the meridians

with emotions. He noted that each meridian was related to a positive and a negative emotion. The heart meridian is identified with anger when negative and with love or forgiveness when positive. The thyroid meridian is associated with depression when negative and with hope and elation when positive, and the liver meridian similarly affects happiness or unhappiness.

Thinking Makes It So

Diamond also demonstrated that life energy is influenced when we think negatively. Stressful circumstances can affect the body. He believes that many of our problems stem from decisions we made in the past that have become incorporated as if part of a predetermined script. Through muscle testing Diamond helps patients determine when the decision was made and the problem began. By treating the meridian points, the energy is then unblocked and change can occur.

The therapeutic power of affirmative thought is a key part of Diamond's approach. He suggests a daily program of positive statements: "I have love," "I reach out with love," "I have forgiveness in my heart," ending with, "My life energy is high. I am in the state of love." As you make each statement, you touch one of the fourteen meridians that correspond to each affirmation. Practicing this each day corrects negative emotional states and promotes a feeling of well-being. Diamond maintains, "Whenever we direct our communication out into the world, whether it be speech, writing, poetry, music or the like, there will always be a greater increase in life energy than if we keep the message to ourselves."

Dr. Roger Callahan's Contribution

Psychologist Roger J. Callahan, Ph.D., was looking for ways to improve his ability to treat his patients when he was introduced to muscle testing. He developed Thought Field Therapy after studying Applied Kinesiology. Thought Field Therapy is the first organized system specifically designed to treat psychological distress by balancing the body's energy system. Dr. Callahan believes that the cause of psychological problems is a perturbation in what he calls the individual's thought field. The disturbance in the thought field causes disruption in the energy system that affects other systems in the body. Callahan discovered that stimulating specific acupuncture points in a particular sequence could eliminate negative feelings.

Callahan went on to treat a large number of people and studied their reactions. He created recipes, called algorithms, consisting of acupuncture points that must be tapped in a distinct order. Each algorithm is designed to treat a specific emotion, such as panic, anxiety, phobia, addictive urges, or anger. Each recipe consists of a different number of points. In TFT the therapist uses muscle testing to determine meridian disturbances and instructs the client to tap acupuncture points in the prescribed sequence to treat psychological problems.

Psychological Reversal

Dr. Harold Saxton Burr showed that the electromagnetic polarities in the body could reverse when serious medical conditions were present. In his book, *Blueprint for Immortality*, he included a study of women with gynecological problems. Of the women with cervical cancer, 96 percent had a negative electrical charge while 95 percent of women with a noncancerous condition had a positive charge. This finding suggests that if the energy polarities are reversed in the body, it is a sign of difficulty or illness.

One of Dr. Callahan's most important additions to this field is the awareness of the phenomenon he calls *Psychological Reversal*. In *PR* when polarities are reversed, psychological problems don't seem to improve no matter how hard the patient works to overcome his problem. Callahan discovered energy points to tap that undo the reversal and allow the TFT treatment to succeed.

Another aspect of Thought Field Therapy is the *Nine Gamut Treatment*. After tapping the energy points of an algorithm, the individual is next instructed to perform nine actions, such as looking down to the right and left, moving the eyes around in a circle, humming a song, and counting out loud, while tapping an energy point on the back of the hand. This exercise is meant to stimulate the left and right hemispheres of the brain in order to balance energy.

Emotional Freedom Techniques (EFT)

Roger Callahan trained many innovative and talented people who went on to create variations of Thought Field Therapy. Some of them began to question the TFT mandate that the order of tapping acupuncture points is essential for a positive outcome. The need to use a different algorithm for each emotional state was challenged too. Some practitioners have found that the process works by touching rather than tapping or even by imagining that tapping is taking place.

One of the most inventive of Callahan's students is Gary Craig, an engineer and personal performance coach. He calls his system Emotional Freedom Techniques or EFT. Craig created a comprehensive formula for tapping, a "one size fits all" treatment in which all the energy meridians are stimulated. This is the only procedure necessary to treat anger, fear, panic, cravings, trauma, guilt, shame, grief, pain, and other emotional problems. With EFT you activate fewer acupuncture points than with TFT. But EFT even gets results without using the Nine Gamut Treatment, which is an integral part of TFT.

Craig also teaches an advanced form of EFT in which people learn to help themselves more efficiently by using intuition to discover which acupuncture points to tap. He found that it is not always necessary to stimulate all the points in the comprehensive formula for success. Through his many workshops, videos, and website, Craig freely shares the EFT process with professionals and the public.

Be Set Free Fast (BSFF)

Be Set Free Fast is what Larry Nims, Ph.D., calls his method. BSFF relies on the idea that unresolved negative emotions and beliefs cause problems. Nims believes that thoughts, feelings, and behavior are affected by subconscious programming. He teaches that all psychological issues are recorded in the subconscious mind, which he calls our "faithful servant." BSFF treats every psychological, physical, or spiritual problem that has emotional roots. Unlike TFT and EFT, BSFF uses an algorithm composed of only three acupuncture points. The user focuses on his problem while affirming that he is eliminating all the sadness, fear, anger or emotional trauma, in all of the roots and the deepest cause of the problem. Muscle testing is also used in BSFF.

BSFF is different from TFT and EFT. Dr. Nims asserts that BSFF is not just a variation of other energy therapies. Those therapies argue that a "perturbation" in the energy field causes the problem, and that all that is needed is to tap on specific energy circuits to balance the energy system. They do not directly address and eliminate the subconscious programming, the belief systems, or the emotional roots of problems.

The very first time you use BSFF, Nims instructs you to contact the subconscious, saying, "Whenever I am treating any problem, I am not only eliminating the emotional roots and deepest cause, but I am also eliminating anything that would make me keep the problem, ever take it back, ever permit it to come back, ever passively allow it to come back, or ever be receptive to it coming back." Nims estimates that up to two thousand emotional roots or unresolved experiences from the past can be resolved simultaneously for each problem when using the BSFF algorithm. A more recent development called Instant BSFF works without tapping points. The subconscious is instructed to automatically carry out the treatment when you say a trigger word or phrase.

Negative Affect Erasing Method (NAEM)

NAEM is a system created by Dr. Fred Gallo, Ph.D., also trained by Dr. Roger Callahan. Gallo treats traumas, phobias, anxiety, depression, and other emotional states with a simple four-point algorithm, which uses points at the "third eye" and the thymus gland, as well as other acupuncture points.

Dr. Gallo's Energy Diagnostic and Treatment Methods or EDxTM teaches how to find the most effective meridian point or cluster of points to alleviate imbalances in the energy system. This approach individualizes treatment and is especially helpful when TFT or EFT algorithms aren't effective. Gallo's approach also deals with correcting the energy disruptions caused by negative core beliefs.

The Future of Energy Psychology

The methods developed by Gary Craig, Larry Nims, Fred Gallo, and others are based on stimulating the body's energy meridians. Their students are creating even more variations of energy-based psychology. Thanks to the wonders of the Internet, information about the latest ideas is shared by thousands of people around the world. Discussion continues about the nature of the bioelectromagnetic qualities of the body and how healing can be facilitated. Energy Psychology conferences are now offered in the United States, Canada, Australia, and Switzerland.

As we proceed in the twenty-first century, emotional problems will be treated more rapidly, efficiently, and permanently because of the expanding knowledge of the body/mind concept and the growing acceptance of the healing powers within. The simplicity of Meridian Therapy techniques offer people a wonderful opportunity to help themselves.

The Meridian Therapy System

Meridian Therapy is the term I have chosen to describe all the various ways of stimulating meridians to heal emotional problems. The system presented in this book blends concepts from each of the approaches that I have just described with ideas from professionals around the world and my own skills as a psychotherapist and teacher. As you use the techniques in this book, you will learn how a simple tapping procedure can relieve fear, stress, anxiety, panic, anger, cravings, pain, and more. Meridian Therapy is so easy you may wonder if it is too good to be true. Try it and find out.

chapter two

Teach Yourself
Meridian Therapy
in Five Simple Steps

You can learn Meridian Therapy in five simple steps and begin using it immediately. Meridian Therapy is so simple even a child can learn it. Seven-year-old Andy explained, "My school bus was late taking me home once, and I was scared. I used tapping to help me, and it worked. It helped me feel a lot better."

To treat yourself, all you have to do is gently tap eight energy points on your face, hands, and upper body while thinking about the thing that is upsetting you. Each point is an acupuncture point related to a specific energy meridian. You will be able to memorize the points in a few minutes. After you learn which energy points to tap, I will teach you how to treat yourself in five simple steps.

• • •

The Basic Points

Start by familiarizing yourself with the eight tapping points. Use two fingers, the index and middle fingers, to tap with.

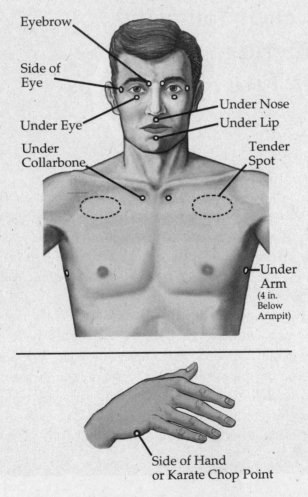

Meridian Therapy Tapping Points

You can tap with either hand and on either side of your face and body. Tap each spot gently but firmly five to ten times in order to stimulate the energy meridians.

The easiest way to memorize the points is to start at the top and work down. If you use your left hand, you will be tracing the letter S, and if you use your right, the letter Z.

Starting Points

Choose one:
- *Karate Chop spot* is the fleshy part on the outside edge of your hand below the little finger.
- *Tender spot* is on your upper chest near the shoulder, which is tender when you rub it.

Remaining Points

- *Eyebrow point* is on the inner ridge of the eyebrow, near the nose.
- *Side of Eye point* is on the bone at the outer corner of the eye.
- *Under the Eye point* is under the middle of the eye but above the cheekbone.
- *Under the Nose point* is directly under the nose and above the upper lip.
- *Under the Lower Lip point* is in the indentation under the lower lip.
- *Under the Collarbone point* is approximately 1 inch below the collarbone and 1 inch off center.
- *Under the Arm point* is approximately 4 inches below the armpit on the side of the body.

Practice tapping these points a few times until you get the knack. In a very short while you will be able to complete the sequence in seconds. It doesn't matter in what order you tap the points. Most people find it easiest to go from top to bottom.

Step One: Target the Problem

Before you start tapping, decide which problem, situation, negative emotion, or unhappy memory you want to address. The first thing that you may think of is your overall problem: sleep disturbance, fear of flying, anxiety about speaking in public, unhappy relationship with X, money worries, smoking problem, chronic headaches, and so forth. You will experience more significant outcomes if you break the problem down into definable aspects and tap each one rather than thinking about the larger picture.

Name the Specific Issues

Focus on individual parts of the problem or particular feelings to produce positive results.

- Instead of "sleep problem," perhaps you want to pin it down to "being wide awake at 4:00 A.M. and can't get back to sleep" or "I toss and turn until midnight."
- Rather than being general about fear of public speaking, focus on the specific presentation you will be giving at work on Wednesday. Make it clear in your mind by picturing the surroundings and the audience.

- What is troublesome about your relationship with X? "I resent X's criticism of my work." "I'm never good enough for X."
- Pinpoint specific money worries: "I'll never have enough money." "I don't know how I'll pay the rent this month." "I'm jealous of my brother's big new house."

Choose individual negative memories.

- The time my teacher embarrassed me in front of the whole class in the third grade
- My grandmother's death
- My gallbladder surgery
- The time I was mugged
- My car accident last summer

Choose a present-day thought or feeling that immediately concerns you.

- I'm afraid I will drink too much at Mary's dinner party.
- I just had a fight with my spouse and am feeling sad.
- I am furious with the car mechanic!
- My child's teacher wants to see me after school. Is he in trouble?
- I have to go for a flu shot, and I'm afraid of needles.
- They are announcing a layoff at work next week, and I am very anxious.
- My in-laws are coming to visit!

If you can't think of something specific, try to see how you are feeling in general. Occasionally I find myself tapping, "I'm grumpy," or, "Something is bothering me, but I don't know what it is." If no words come, become aware of any discomfort in your body. Perhaps there is a lump in your throat, heaviness in your chest, tears behind your eyes, or butterflies in your stomach. These can be very important and useful signs. Start with what you feel.

Step Two:
Rate Your Feelings from Zero to Ten

Once you have determined what you want to treat, ask yourself how upset you feel right now. Rate the intensity of your negative emotion or pain on a scale from zero to ten. Ten means it feels intensely unpleasant. Zero does not mean happy; it means free of negative charge, a neutral feeling. The goal is to follow the Meridian Therapy procedure until you reduce the negative sensation to zero.

If you aren't comfortable with the numerical rating scale, take a piece of paper and put an X on the top to indicate your emotional state at the beginning. Put a zero on the bottom to indicate your goal. After each round of tapping, tune in to your level of discomfort, and see if anything is changing. What is your level now? Did it go up, go down, or stay the same? Put a dot or an X on your paper to show where the negative feeling is.

This rating system doesn't have to be exact. It just needs to give you some idea whether you are extremely emotional, moderately annoyed, anxious, scared, or mildly upset. As you complete a round of Meridian Therapy your negative emotions or physical pain will change and usually decrease or disappear. It can happen gradually or in seconds.

The rating system will help you become aware of what is happening. Because Meridian Therapy works so rapidly, some people doubt its efficacy and report that they weren't really feeling bad to begin with. I have had numerous clients say, "I can't believe this!" as their fears or traumatic memories lessen. Yes, it is hard to believe if you have never experienced it before. Keep track by writing the numbers down so you will have proof and can measure the change.

Step Three: Say the Affirmation

The affirmation helps you to face your problem while at the same time reinforcing self-acceptance. By using the affirmation, you maintain that although you suffer from a negative emotion or difficult condition, you are not the problem.

The first part is very simple to do. Either tap the Karate Chop spot or rub the Tender spot on the upper chest vigorously. It doesn't matter which hand you use. While you are tapping or rubbing, speak in a strong and expressive voice.

Say three times with feeling: *Even though I have this problem, I deeply and completely accept myself!*

Create your own version of this affirmation to make it more meaningful. Describe the situation or feeling rather than use the generic phrase "this problem." Here are some samples.

- Even though I am angry with Bill and wish he would go away, I know that God loves me.
- Even though I pigged out on ice cream last night, I deeply accept myself as a good person.
- Even though I am afraid to talk in front of a group, I profoundly love and accept myself.
- Even though I don't want to go to the dentist because I may find out that I need a painful root canal, I accept myself today.

Many people report that just saying the affirmation aloud three times with feeling has an immediate positive effect on their unhappiness.

Bigger and Better Affirmations

When you expand the affirmation and tell more details about the issue, the result is both creative and very powerful. All the while you tap the Karate Chop spot or rub the Tender spot, talk about the problem in greater detail. Affirm your own part in it and forgive yourself. It might sound like this:

"Even though I have this problem [name your problem], I love myself and forgive myself for anything I might have done to contribute to it. And I love and forgive anyone else who may have contributed to it."

"Even though I have this problem and I don't really know if I want to let go of it, and I feel guilty and ashamed because I should let go of it, and I feel like an awful person for keeping it, I forgive and accept myself."

"Even though I want to quit smoking but don't want to give up the pleasure because it is all I have left since I gave up alcohol, and I resent all those people who are trying to make me quit, I fully accept and love myself."

No I Don't!

"But I don't accept and love myself," you may say. Think up a phrase you can affirm. Some people say things like, "I am doing my best just for today," " I am a child of God," or, "I am a decent human being." Another option is to make this paradoxical statement and see what occurs when you do a round of tapping: "Even though I don't accept and love myself, I completely and profoundly accept myself."

Step Four:
Follow the Tapping Sequence

After you say the affirmation three times, tap each of the additional seven points with your index and third finger. Gently tap five to ten times on each spot: Eyebrow, Side of Eye, Under Eye, Under Nose, Under Lip, Under Collarbone, Under Arm. Then take a deep breath and let it out. Notice your level of disturbance. Did it go down? By how much? Keep track of this after every round of tapping.

Use a Reminder

The words that come after "even though" in the affirmation are a statement of the problem, emotion, or memory you want to treat. If you name your problem as you tap, you will get a better result because focused thoughts amplify your intentions. Say a reminder phrase once at each tapping point. You can say it out loud or to yourself.

"I am afraid to go to the dentist because I might find out I need a root canal" can be shortened to "dental fear," "tooth fear," or "root canal" as a reminder.

"I pigged out on ice cream" can turn to "pigged out," "binge," or "ice cream."

All you need is a key word or phrase to remind you of your problem. Once you know what the problem is, all you have to say is "Bill," "my boss," "Vietnam," "migraine." Or you can choose to call it "this problem" or "this memory," or "the pain."

Use your own words! Say exactly what you mean. Describe the problem in a way you can connect with emotionally. Occasionally you won't know exactly what the problem is or what particular feeling you are experiencing. As long as you know something is disturbing you, you can tap. I have tapped, "Whatever this is that is bothering me," "I feel blah," and "I'm down in the dumps."

Do I Have to Accentuate the Negative?

The most common complaint I get from my clients is that they don't want to speak negative phrases or identify themselves with a problem. However, it is necessary to attune to the energy disturbance in order to treat it, the same way you would tune in a radio station. Reminding yourself of the problem will enable you to zero in on the energy disturbance more efficiently so healing can take place.

As your level of disturbance decreases, change your reminder phrase to reflect what is happening. You can say "remaining anger" to denote that transformation is taking place. Some of the anger is gone, so you are now dealing with what remains. Another way to reassure yourself that something is happening is to say "releasing anger." You may even choose "anger at a five," if your disturbance level has dropped from an eight to a five.

Speaking the reminder word or phrase keeps your mind on the process. Even though you are talking out loud, you can think faster than you can talk. You will frequently notice that new thoughts, understandings, emotions, physical sensations, or memories come to mind during the tapping sequence or just afterward.

Watch What Happens

Maybe you are doing a round of tapping in which you remind yourself that you are angry with Tom because he isn't answering your phone calls. A feeling of sadness may replace that anger as you become aware that Tom recently lost his mother and has a lot on his mind. That may be why he is acting irritable or forgetful. When you go back to check your anger, you will discover that it has changed. It may feel more like mild resentment or it may be totally gone.

As one feeling or thought fades another may pop up. Follow the flow. Use the new thought or feeling as your reminder in round two. You may begin with a craving for a cigarette and, as you tap, you realize that you don't want to give up the pleasure of smoking. Begin the second round with the thought "I don't want to give it up." Perhaps as you tap you feel a lump in your throat. Begin the next round by focusing on the sensation and saying "lump in throat."

Valerie Discovers Compassion

Revise your reminding phrase to reflect the process of change. Here is an example of Valerie's process. She was annoyed with her husband, Phil, because he liked to take long naps in his free time and wasn't available for other activities. She started out concentrating on her anger about the naps. On the next round she felt sad for Phil because he had his own problems, so she said "this sadness" when she tapped. She went on from there to realize that she felt some guilt about being a homemaker while he was stuck in a job he didn't really like in order to provide for the family. The third round she said "guilt." With each round of Meridian Therapy, another new awareness of the issue sprang to mind. Valerie kept changing her reminder until she felt finished with her anger.

Even if you start to wander to other issues, keep coming back to the original problem and rate your level of disturbance. Repeat the tapping until you get to zero.

Step Five: Take Stock

When you complete a round of tapping, stop, take a deep breath, and let it out. Notice what just occurred. Think of your problem. Has your level of discomfort gone down, gone up, remained the same? While you were tapping, did any new thoughts or sensations come up? Did a memory pop into your mind? Did you have an insight into your problem that changes things, as Valerie did?

If the rating of the emotional intensity of your problem is lower than when you started, repeat steps four and five again and again, as necessary, until you reach zero. Keep in mind that zero means you feel neutral about your problem, not that you feel happy. It is not necessary to repeat the affirmation unless the level of discomfort is not dropping or you change to a new topic or problem.

Here are some examples of what happened to people I counseled when they used Meridian Therapy for their problems.

Alice Quickly Finds a Solution

Alice tried the Five Simple Steps and was amazed at the speedy result. When she found a $29 late penalty on her credit card bill Alice was incensed because she had mailed her payment so it would arrive before the due date. She rated her anger eight. After the first round of tapping it was five, then two, and finally zero. At that point she reached for the phone to complain. As a result, the credit card company immediately credited her with the $29. The entire process took only three minutes.

Cynthia Releases the Past

Cynthia discovered that memories appeared as she tapped about a marriage problem. Cynthia and Barry had been married for ten years. Cynthia was treating herself for anger toward Barry because he often made promises he didn't keep. She was livid. "He has let me down so often that he has destroyed my trust in him," she said.

As she tapped, she remembered the times her father had done the same thing. When she was seven, Dad promised her a horse but didn't follow through. Many other promises never materialized. Cynthia switched from tapping about

Barry to tapping about her father's betrayal of her trust. When that reached zero, she returned to her thoughts and feelings about Barry. She was surprised that she was now able to see him in a new light and not as an incarnation of her father.

Jerry's Aha!

Insight changed the way Jerry perceived his problem. Jerry, a forty-three-year-old man, kept changing jobs. He had trouble getting along with people and usually blamed his troubles on everyone else. As he tapped Jerry remembered how much he had hated his old job and the coworkers who gave him a hard time. After three rounds he came to a surprising realization. "I wasn't much of a team player. I often came to work late or didn't show up at all. I was using drugs too much at the time. My attitude was negative and surly. No wonder they didn't like me," he said. His hostility immediately faded, as he understood how his own behavior had created his problem.

Alice, Cynthia, and Jerry were delighted with their outcomes after less than ten minutes of Meridian Therapy. You can be, too! Continue to follow the Five Simple Steps until your anger, fear, panic, anxiety or craving is gone, or you have reached a solution to the problem and feel at peace.

Test Yourself

When you think all the negative charge has disappeared from your problem, test yourself by trying with all your might to get the anger, fear, or anxiety back. Don't be afraid to try this. If anything negative remains use the Five Simple Steps sequence again. Keep retesting until you feel neutral.

If you are dealing with an event or memory that was unpleasant, close your eyes and rerun the memory in your mind as if it were a movie. At the first sign of remaining discomfort, stop and tap that scene. Then rerun it again. Keep doing this until you can see the movie from start to finish without reacting.

Another way to test yourself is to say something out loud that a few minutes ago created intense feelings or tears. Notice how you feel when you loudly say:

"He raped me and no one helped me."

"I hate her!"

"I am terrified of speaking in front of the group tomorrow."

"That car almost hit me as I was changing lanes. I could have died."

"My father didn't love me."

If you can say the inflammatory sentence free of a negative emotional reaction, you are at zero. There is no more to do.

Frequently Asked Questions

Q: How many minutes does it take to give myself a Meridian Therapy treatment?

A: A treatment can be completed in one or two sequences of tapping that take several minutes or longer. When you want to eliminate negative emotions like fear, anxiety, and anger about a designated incident, one treatment may resolve it. You may feel relief in one minute, after just one or two rounds. Complicated issues may bring up memories or new thoughts and take longer to resolve.

Some problems can take many hours to deal with. You will need many Meridian Therapy sessions to address complex problems like traumatic memories, compulsions, or procrastination because new aspects of the issue arise as you continue to apply Meridian Therapy. Treat yourself once or many times a day. You are finished when your discomfort is gone or you are at a place that feels comfortable to you.

Q: Should I use Meridian Therapy daily or occasionally?
A: Some people use Meridian Therapy, from time to time, to deal with strong negative emotions or immediate challenges. Once you know the points by heart you will be able to use it on the spur of the moment or to resolve long-term problems. Some of the ways people have benefited are: tapping when you wake from a bothersome dream, treating after-dinner heartburn, relieving a headache, calming a fearful child, and removing a fear.

How Does Your Garden Grow?

Tap frequently during the day when you are dealing with a problem or relationship, as Jane did (see opposite). It only takes a few minutes to treat yourself. Using Meridian Therapy every day to take the edge off your stress is like weed whacking. Don't feed your emotional weeds. Nip them in the bud with daily tapping. The more you tap, the more you will remember to tap. You don't have to sweat the small stuff—just tap it away.

Jane Almost Loses Her Job

Knowing how to tap came in handy for Jane, whose marriage problems were upsetting her so much that she often missed work or couldn't concentrate. Her boss told her that her job was on the line. One morning Jane had a fight with her husband before she left for work. She was so distraught that she was considering going home. Jane went into the ladies room, where she could have privacy, and tapped her rage and frustration. She was soon calm enough to go back to her desk and was able to keep her mind on her job.

Q: How will I know if I am doing it correctly?

A: Specific feelings of fear, anxiety, anger, guilt, shame, and craving will disappear. Sad or frightening memories will no longer affect you. They will become neutralized, as if you are looking at photos in an album. You will see problems in a new light and find new solutions that feel appropriate.

Q: What will I experience as I tap?

A: You may have different feelings and responses every time you tap. Some of the common reactions to Meridian Therapy are relaxation, feeling energy in your body, sighing, giggling, sadness, anger, crying, remembering, understanding, release, and relief.

Changing the Subject

When new thoughts, memories, or feelings seem to interrupt, they are called "aspects." You may think you aren't doing Meridian Therapy correctly because your mind keeps coming up with new ideas or memories as you tap. Aspects are signs of other material that relates to your problem and is coming to your attention. Aspects are like the branches of a tree. There may be many, and each branch may have little twigs. Notice the different aspects that came up as Donna dealt with a sleep problem.

Donna Discovers Aspects

Donna was tired all the time. "It's hard to get myself to go to bed. I have trouble falling asleep and staying asleep," she said. This is what happened when I guided Donna through the Five Simple Steps for her sleep problem.

Round one: Tap "my sleep problem."
Awareness: After the birth of my baby I was very depressed and couldn't sleep for days at a time.

Round two: Tap " birth of baby."
Awareness: My marriage was in trouble at that time.

Round three: Tap "troubled marriage."
Awareness: I am suddenly thinking about how I am afraid of the dark.

Round four: Tap "afraid of the dark."
Awareness: I remember I was molested by a neighbor when I was small.

Round five: Tap "molest memory."
Awareness: I told my parents.

Round six: Tap "molest upset."
Awareness: Nothing new.

Round seven: Tap "remaining molest memory."
Awareness: I remember that I would wake up during the night and feel all alone while the others slept. It was dark and scary.

Round eight: Tap "awake and alone."
Awareness: I am feeling better.

Round nine: Tap "remaining memory."
Awareness: I feel OK.

At this point Donna tried to remember the molestation again. She now felt neutral about it. No upsetting emotion remained. It seemed like a good stopping point. After this session her sleep started to improve significantly.

What to Expect

One of the pluses of Meridian Therapy is that, in an emergency, it can be employed on the spot. That is what happened to Barbara, a frequent flyer afraid of turbulence. She was able to treat herself during an especially rocky airline flight and, thereafter, made many more such trips without the fear recurring.

Some problems are multifaceted. Meridian Therapy will help peel the layers away. As one aspect of a problem or memory is dealt with another often surfaces. Don't give up if relief doesn't come immediately. Continue tapping until you reach a zero for each part. It is up to you how long and how often you wish to use Meridian Therapy for a particular subject.

Conditions like depression and compulsion take a longer time to work with. Tap at least ten times a day for one minute for the best outcome. Continuing life problems won't disappear in moments. Support groups, twelve-step groups, and psychotherapy are helpful when tackling major self-defeating patterns. Once you know how to do Meridian Therapy, it can become an important part of your problem-solving skills.

Take Baby Steps

Begin slowly as you get used to tapping your troubles away. Many people want to plunge in and address their most important or most painful problem. Looking into problems of addiction and compulsion, traumatic memories, depression, and procrastination will bring up many aspects or roots. First become adept at using Meridian Therapy before you tackle these intricate topics. Later in this book I will discuss how to work with more serious problems and issues that affect your life. Hold off tackling sexual or physical abuse memories or specific post-traumatic stress symptoms until you are more experienced. If you are already in psychotherapy about these experiences, check with your doctor or therapist about your readiness to address these memories by yourself.

For starters choose something in your life that, when you think about it, produces a level of discomfort of five or less. Stay away from the tens until you are more proficient. Practice with the milder memories, fears, or angers until you feel competent. Select a subject that is concrete and specific. You will then be able to experience the drop in your negative energy clearly. Instead of thinking about your unhappiness at work, limit your focus to your dissatisfaction with a coworker who stays on the phone making personal calls, leaving you to do his work. Experiment by taking a food, cigarette, or glass of wine or beer that you want but are telling yourself you shouldn't have, and tap on that one instance of desire.

Earmark one worry you have right now: an unexpected bill, anger with another person, fear or anxiety about something that is about to happen now or in the next few days. You may be in pain as you read this. Try the Five Simple Steps for an ache in your shoulder, a headache, or another specific physical sensation. Chapter 11: Boost Your Physical Health and Well-Being, will tell you more about this.

Now you are ready to put Meridian Therapy into action!

Five Simple Steps Summary

1. Choose a problem.
2. Tune in and rate the intensity of your negative feeling from zero to ten.
3. State the affirmation three times while tapping the Karate Chop spot or rubbing the Tender spot.
4. Tap the remaining energy points as you speak a reminder word or phrase.
5. Take a deep breath and take stock. What is the rating now? Notice any new thoughts, feelings, or memories. Repeat steps four and five until you reach zero or the problem is resolved.

chapter three

Tap Dancing: Seven More Ways to Use Meridian Therapy

Once you become familiar with the basics of Meridian Therapy, you will notice that you can do it quickly. Soon you will be able perform the Five Simple Steps in less than one minute. You might be wondering if you can improve on Meridian Therapy or "do your own thing." The answer is "Yes." Thousands of people all over the world are using Meridian Therapy successfully. Many are also playing with the possibilities for making the technique more efficient or more fun to do. Here are seven creative shortcuts and innovative variations that you may want to try.

1. Narrative Meridian Therapy

You have a problem that you want to talk about but no one is around. Maybe you had a dream the other night that is still on your mind, and you wish you could understand what it means. Sometimes your problem is too personal to trust to another, yet you are puzzled about how to resolve it. These are good times to use the Narrative Meridian Therapy method.

Narrative Meridian Therapy is simply talking out loud to yourself while you tap the energy points. It also works if you say the words silently to yourself, thinking them in your head. Keep tapping round after round. Say a new sentence at each energy point, and keep talking to yourself without stopping, until you are satisfied with the result.

You will want to be totally honest with yourself to get the best results. Use your own words. It's all right to admit feelings and thoughts you might be ashamed of if others could hear you. It's OK to use curse words, if that is how you feel. Pretending that things are fine when they aren't or telling yourself that your rage or fear is childish keeps you from clearing the negativity contributing to your unease and unhappiness. These negative thoughts and feelings are like pus in a wound. Clean them out!

Carol's Cussing

Carol was furious with her family. She would be fairly restrained when talking to a friend. Then she would say, "I hate them for what they did. I wish I never had to see them again." What she really was thinking sounded very different: "I wish I had an Uzi and could mow them down. I would like to annihilate every one of those *%$#@ people. They don't deserve to live after what they did to me!" Of course Carol wouldn't act out her rage, but she felt better after venting her feelings while tapping. After a minute or two the anger dissipated. Then Carol felt great sadness both for herself and for the emotionally troubled people who brought her up.

Avoiding a Fight

One evening I received a call from Shawna, an attractive woman in her forties, who was at her twenty-three-year-old boyfriend's apartment. She was very upset but couldn't figure out why. She knew that he hadn't done or said anything to disturb her, but the feeling wouldn't go away. Shawna knew that if she let her agitation remain and grow, she would start a fight with him for no reason. I instructed her to go to a private place and use the narrative approach.

Tapping and talking out loud to herself released what was really bothering her. Her fears and negative thoughts were about being older than her boyfriend. She worried that he would eventually want someone younger. As she tapped she realized that her maturity and intelligence were what made her such an interesting and fascinating partner. All dread dissolved as she tapped. She was then able to be loving and happy in a genuine way, without effort.

Tracy's Night Terror

Tracy, a sixty-year-old professional woman, was upset because she was waking up at 3:00 A.M. with a terror about dying. This happened a few nights in a row. She began to worry about going to bed the next night. As she talked and tapped it sounded something like this:

- "I don't like these feelings of terror. I am afraid."
- "Uh-oh, next week is my sixtieth birthday. Sixty, that's old."
- "This aging thing is awful. I don't want to get old."
- "Getting old means becoming invisible. I will fade away."

- "People won't take me seriously and know who I am."
- "When people know who I am it makes me feel alive."
- "I am an achiever. I want to keep it that way."
- "Fame fades. Where are all the famous people from my youth now?"
- "Is this what it is all about, being known and recognized?"
- "But it's too late in my life. Time and opportunity have passed me by."
- "It's never too late. Who knows what else I will do in my life!"
- "I feel regret, regret, regret" (tapped the same word on all points).
- "I'm remembering all the men who were my contemporaries."
- "They are 'out there' leading things, being renowned."
- "Anger, anger, anger" (tapped the same word on all points).
- "My generation couldn't achieve like those men. We were pressured to become wives and mothers first."
- "Too late! You only get one chance and I blew it."
- "Nonsense."
- "I feel sad, sad, sad, sad" (tapped the same word on all points).
- "I am through with this old stuff. I don't need it anymore."
- "I feel better now."

Tracy felt free of her unhappiness after less than five minutes, using the narrative method. Her sleep improved, and she stopped thinking about the past and got on with new projects.

When to Talk to Yourself

Narrative Meridian Therapy works best with a specific feeling or issue that can be narrowly pinpointed. It is also good to use in an emergency, as Shawna did. If you try to talk to yourself about a global problem like depression, compulsion, or trauma, you may find yourself stuck, going around and around in a negative loop. When that happens stop using the Narrative approach, and go back to the Five Simple Steps of Meridian Therapy.

2. Two-Handed Tapping

Some people feel more comfortable using both hands to tap the same points on the left and right sides simultaneously. John reported that he felt more balanced using two-handed tapping and got a sense of greater resolution. "It just feels right," he said. Acupressure practitioners maintain that it balances the yin and yang energy. Try both one-handed and two-handed Meridian Therapy and compare.

3. Mental Tapping

Joseph can't tap because he is a quadriplegic. He suffers constant pain and frequent muscle spasms. He discovered that when he clearly imagined tapping each energy point, he could diminish the pain. Joseph enjoys having some control over his condition.

Use Your Imagination

You can use Mental Tapping too when you're feeling strong emotions but can't get away to a private place to tap. Tap in your imagination. Think of your problem. Go through the sequence by putting your attention on each Meridian Therapy point and holding it there for a few seconds. Picture your fingers tapping each point. Imagine the feeling on your skin. Say "tap, tap, tap" to yourself. Experiment and find what works best for you.

My friend Julia was having dinner in a noisy restaurant with a friend before going to a play. She put her hand up to her ear to adjust her button hearing aid and discovered that it was gone. Julia panicked. The hearing aids she wears are very expensive and take a while to replace. She didn't have time to go home to see if she had dropped it there or lost it in the dress store where she had tried on clothing that afternoon. As her anxiety mounted, she thought of Meridian Therapy but didn't want to do it in front of her dinner partner. She simply used her imagination. After only one sequence the panic was gone. She went to the theater and had an enjoyable evening. What a relief it was to find the hearing aid on the floor of the bedroom when she got home.

Mental tapping can be done anywhere, any time. You can do it in a meeting, on a plane, in a doctor's office, or at a party. You can do it alone or with others present.

4. The Body Knows

Tension in your body may represent stress in your life. Your body is telling you something, and you can learn to decode the message. Negative emotions often show up as physical discomfort. You may not be aware you are feeling angry, yet you grind your teeth in your sleep. Distress in the body can lead to muscle or joint pain. Focus on the physical sensation rather than words that describe a problem. Begin with a pain in your neck, shoulder, or back, heaviness in your chest, or a lump in your throat. Use the Five Simple Steps, saying, "Even though my lower back is hurting, I completely accept myself."

After the first round of Meridian Therapy notice what has happened. Has the discomfort lessened or disappeared? Has it moved elsewhere? If it has lessened, keep tapping until it is gone. If it has moved to another part of your body, tap that new sensation. Follow the pain as it moves to different places in your body. After each round, notice the changes. Keep this up until the pain is gone.

As you stimulate the energy meridians to resolve a specific negative feeling like anger, anxiety, guilt, or shame, or to heal a traumatic memory, the words may go away and be replaced by a distinct sensation. That's OK. Don't try to put it into words, just tap as you feel the discomfort. You may even go back and forth between emotional feelings, thoughts, and body sensations. Follow the Five Simple Steps until you feel neutral, and the tensions, pains, or tightness are gone.

5. Touch and Breathe

Another approach that may appeal to you is called Touch and Breathe. TAB is a gentle substitute for tapping created by Dr. John Diepold. Use Meridian Therapy as described in the Five Simple Steps. Instead of tapping, gently touch the energy point and take one or more normal breaths with each touch. This technique is especially helpful for people with arthritis or other problems that make tapping on the face or body uncomfortable.

6. Daily Workout

Going to the gym every day to keep fit is a popular pastime. Many of us take vitamins daily for our health. I practice Meridian Therapy every day as a mental health preventative. With the Daily Workout you can tap your troubles away before they can grow and fester into a major problem. I prefer to tap in the morning to remove the cobwebs of care that can ruin my day. Tap at any time that is best for you. Tap in the shower. Tap before you get out of bed or before you go to bed at night. Tap before you start your car or while it is warming up. Tap at red lights. I prefer to tap while I take my daily walk.

I Didn't Know It Was Helping

One November a few years ago I hurt my foot and wasn't able to walk for exercise while it healed. Since I do my Daily Meridian Therapy Workout during my walk, I stopped tapping regularly. I thought nothing of it and seemed to be getting along all right. Although the weather in California was beautiful that December I seemed to have winter in my heart. I was surly and irritable. I kept telling my friends I was having a "Bah Humbug Christmas." All through the month my husband would ask, "What is wrong with you?"

As December ended my doctor allowed me to resume

exercise. Within three days of walking and tapping my mood transformed. My anger and negativity melted. It was obvious to me that doing the Daily Meridian Therapy Workout had kept me on an even keel emotionally. I felt good again and hadn't attributed my sense of well-being to Meridian Therapy until I noticed the change.

Create Your Own Workout

Daily Meridian Therapy can last one or two minutes or longer. The time you take to change your mood and feel energized will be different each day and reflect the ups and downs in your life. I suggest that you divide your daily regime into these three parts. However, you can do whatever works best for you as long as you do it every day.

Part One: Feel Fit

First, focus on physical well-being. As you begin, take stock of how you feel. Are you sleepy or tired due to a poor night's sleep? Do you feel dyspeptic after eating spicy foods? Any aches or pains? Tap on all unpleasant sensations until you clear them. You don't have to use a rating because you will know when the discomfort has disappeared.

Part Two: Today's Worries

Next, think about the problems that are on your mind, things that you are worried, fearful, or angry about.

- Uh-oh, it is time to pay your taxes—and you didn't expect to owe this much.

- One of your children is starting to act rebellious, and you are so upset your gut is in an uproar because you are worried that he is on drugs.
- Your boss passed you over for a special assignment and gave it to someone not as qualified. You are steamed.
- You are frantic because your cat is missing.
- The plumber said he would come at 8:00 A.M. and it is now 10:00 A.M.

As you review these issues you will notice that you are in touch with your anger, sadness, fear, or worry and can rate the negative emotional charge from zero to ten. These are the things that are "in your face" today. Take each one and tap until you have reached zero and feel calm. As you stimulate the energy meridians, solutions may come to mind, or realizations abut what action needs to be taken. A sense of peace will come over you.

I Don't Know What's Wrong

If you can't think of anything specific, perhaps you are just feeling jittery or down in the dumps. Tap those feelings, saying, "Even though I feel down in the dumps, I completely and profoundly accept myself." After a few rounds ideas may come to mind revealing what is really going on underneath.

Do you hide what you are worried about from yourself because you are ashamed to admit you have certain feelings? Part of you knows it isn't "nice" to feel envy or jealousy, yet you sometimes do. Admitting you are so angry with someone that you would like to hurt them can be scary. You know you would never actually do it, but even thinking about it causes guilt. You may think you have pushed it out of your mind, but you haven't, so you might as well tap it away for good. One of the wonderful things about Meridian Therapy is that you can keep all the negative thoughts in the privacy of your own head while treating yourself.

Part Three: Long-Term Projects

Finally, treat your long-term projects. These are situations, behavior, chronic illnesses, or problems that won't go away in a few minutes. One common complaint is waking in the middle of the night and not being able to go back to sleep. The next morning you feel sleepy or cranky, but you can't recreate the feeling of frustration of lying in bed wide awake at 4:00 A.M. Simply remember it and tap on the thought of waking up in the middle of the night. You don't need to rate it from zero to ten.

Use Daily Meridian Therapy as a continuing treatment. Create a reminder phrase that fits your chronic situation. "Waking at night," "nighttime misery," "I can't sleep," or "this sleep problem" are different versions of the same thing. Find the phrase that has meaning for you. Tap three to five rounds each day and trust the process.

Anyone who suffers from depression knows that even with powerful antidepressants, the problem doesn't go away immediately. Meridian Therapy is a wonderful adjunct to other treatments for depression. Daily tapping can change your mood. Call it "depression" or describe specific aspects of what you feel: "too tired to go out," "hopeless and helpless," "I'm never going to feel good." Be persistent, and you will notice results.

Treat Addiction Daily

Addicts and those battling other compulsive behavior need to use Meridian Therapy every day. Tap as you name the general problem: "addiction," "my problem," "overeating," "using," "drinking," "sugar cravings," or "I can't have just one." Tap about "loss of control," "fear of loss of control," "what I did yesterday," or even "I'll never get over this problem." Keep it simple. Tap for as long as you like. You may be surprised to find you don't want to use Meridian Therapy at all and conveniently forget to tap or find excuses to keep from practicing tapping. If you notice you are resisting, tap while you shout, "I don't want to tap!"

Knowing that you feel powerless over a substance or behavior is just the tip of the iceberg. Make a list of all the other people, places, and situations in your life you feel powerless to change. Use Meridian Therapy, choosing one at a time. Cravings arise from frustration and anger at not being able to control everyone and everything in your life. Apply Meridian Therapy to deal with feelings of powerlessness related to a spouse, children, parents, coworkers, the government, and God. Address other things you cannot change, such as your age, body type, height, skin color, or sex.

Keep It Up

Daily Meridian Therapy need not take long, although some days you will have more on your mind than others. You don't have to tap all three categories every day. Tailor the method to suit your available time and what is going on in your life. As you practice, day by day, you will feel better and better.

7. Speed It Up with a Shortcut

By now you know that you may be able to do a round of Meridian Therapy in less than a minute. If you eliminate tapping the Karate Chop spot or Tender spot and the affirmation, and tap only the remaining seven points, you will shorten it even more. Sometimes you won't be able to take the time to do more than a few seconds of tapping. Use this abbreviated version and you will see results.

The Super Shortcut

After applying Meridian Therapy for a while, you may notice that there is one point that seems to promote dramatic change or feels most satisfying when you stimulate it. When I introduce the energy points to my clients, I sometimes have to remind them to stop tapping under the collarbone or under the arm, for example, because it feels so good they don't seem to notice they are still tapping there. When you don't have time to do the Five Simple Steps, tap your special point. If you don't have a special point, ask your creative unconscious to guess what point would help. This is the "Super Shortcut."

Frequently Asked Questions

Q: How can I help a baby or someone very ill who can't tap themselves?

A: Use surrogate tapping. A surrogate is a stand-in for another. When we share energy in the same space and have positive regard, one person can tap in place of another. The best example of this is shown in the bond between parent and child. When a baby is cranky, the parent can cradle the child and tap while speaking for the child. The person tapped for will benefit the same as by treating herself.

Marianne used surrogate tapping for her husband's snoring. She said, "I've stopped his snoring several times by tapping on myself, while visualizing that he is tapping on himself. I think I am my husband and say, 'Even though I am making these dreadful noises I deeply and completely accept myself.' Usually before I finish two rounds he slowly quiets and stops. He rarely snores at all anymore."

Q: When I tap by myself I don't get the same effect as when I am with my therapist. Am I doing it wrong?
A: You are not doing it wrong. However, many people report a difference. During a counseling session my clients often sigh deeply or giggle when the energy shifts. They experience a noticeable change. Some report that they don't get quite the same release when they work by themselves at home. Regardless, rest assured that Meridian Therapy will still give you great results when you use it on your own.

There appears to be something useful about two people working together. There is a living connection between us that enhances what is going on. In science it is now known that the intention of a scientist can influence the outcome of an experiment. The positive energy radiated by a caring professional, friend, or family member has an effect on the other person. You may want to ask someone you trust to sit near you, in a state of mutuality and support. That special other can hold a positive attitude toward you while you tap or can tap along with you. Notice what happens.

Join the Tapping Revolution!

The seven variations I have described in this chapter are only a beginning. Try them out. Discover which ones work best for you. Meridian Therapy is flexible, so experiment with your own versions and share your discoveries. Now you are ready to learn to tap away stress and negative emotions in the next chapter.

Part Two

The Meridian Therapy Solution to Persistent Problems

chapter four

Tap Away Stress and Negative Emotions

In the movie *Annie*, Little Orphan Annie sings, "The sun will come out tomorrow. . . . It's only a day away." If your days are spent waiting for tomorrow to be better, you are wasting your todays. Some people seem to be more resilient than others, but we all have off days due to stress, anger, anxiety, guilt, grief, or depression, emotions common to all of us. When you use Meridian Therapy daily, you will be able to keep negative feelings to a minimum and enjoy a cheerier outlook today and every day.

Stress, the Number-One Problem

According to *Time* magazine, stress is America's number-one health problem. The National Safety Council estimates that one million employees are absent on an average workday because of stress-related problems. Stress results from a biochemical reaction, the fight-or-flight adrenaline rush that readies the body for short-term challenges. Our lives are filled with stressful moments. When you don't know how to relax between tough situations and your tension level never goes down, serious physical and psychological damage can occur. The vast majority of our visits to primary care physicians are stress-related.

Not all stress is bad. The pressure to win at sports, the excitement of travel, winning the lottery, or getting married also put a strain on our constitution. There is no way to avoid stress, but you can learn to manage it. Some of us are born able to be more upbeat than the rest. A study done by the University of Minnesota indicates that as much as 50 percent of a person's tendency to be happy is inherited. But that leaves 50 percent that we can do something about!

The Ingredients of Stress

What do you really mean when you say you are under stress? Some days it seems like a struggle to feel good. We think, "Look at what my job, spouse, kids, the government, or the weather is doing to me." Some of us want to fight back while others would rather retreat to a desert island. The fight-or-flight reaction means you are feeling either anger or fear. No one is really doing anything threatening to your life unless he has a knife or a gun. You create anger or fear through your reactions to the aspects of your life, your beliefs about what is happening. When you use Meridian Therapy you can tap away that fear or anger. If you can't name what you are feeling, but you know you feel stress, you can use the Five Simple Steps, affirming, "Even though I feel stressed, I totally accept myself."

I recommend using Meridian Therapy while waiting at red lights. If you don't drive, take a moment to tap away your stress each time you wash your hands or before each meal. Simply tap one or two rounds while using the reminder phrase "my stress," or "releasing any stress I have now." You will be "Weed Whacking," lessening the tension at work in your body and keeping your stress level down.

Take a Deep Breath

You may be so used to living under tension that you aren't even aware it's there. My favorite test for stress is the Breath Constriction Test. If you are feeling uptight because of physical or emotional stress, the body tightens, and you may experience a knot in your stomach, neck, or shoulders. Your restricted breathing is the indicator that you are stressed. Do this exercise one or more times a day to instantly let go of stress even though you may not know what is bothering you.

1. Take a deep breath.
2. Rate the depth and pleasure of the breath as Excellent, Good, Fair, or Poor.
3. If your rating is less than Excellent, tap the Karate Chop spot or rub the Tender Spot and say, "Even though my breath is constricted, I completely accept myself."
4. Tap the remaining seven energy points saying, " releasing constriction."
5. Take a deep breath and rate it again.

Keep doing steps one to five until you are breathing wonderfully.

As you do the Breath Constriction Test, awareness of specific worries may appear. You can then tap each one until you feel relaxed.

Anger Gets a Bad Rap

Anger is the result of the buildup of energy that accumulates when your body, property, or self-image is threatened. When someone or something gets in the way of what you want you may feel fear or frustration. The body mobilizes for action, heart rate speeds up, adrenaline output increases, but nothing happens. It is as if you assembled troops for a skirmish and called off the battle without telling the troops where to go or what to do. The result is anger. The stored energy may then seek another outlet or target, such as the body, the self, or some other person or object.

When you were growing up, if you were told to "stop it" when you got angry, where did the anger go? Did you push it down and put on a happy face or allow it to smolder like the embers of a fire, just below the surface? Many of us were told that anger was unacceptable. Did you learn that anger was bad and decide that you were bad because you were angry? It is impossible to go through life without feeling angry, yet how you express your animosity may hurt yourself or others. Those who stuff it down often turn to alcohol, drugs, food, and other substances to soothe the rage. Binges are temper tantrums. Most or all of the anger is turned inward.

Where Does the Anger Go?

This is what happened to Virginia, a problem drinker who usually had trouble expressing her anger. She would feel the rage but pour herself a glass or two of wine rather than express it. One evening she discovered that she had been "slammed." Her long-distance telephone carrier was switched, without her permission, to a company that could charge her a higher rate. She felt powerless and enraged. She was furious! Although it was time for bed, she was wide awake and craving a large glass of wine. Before she opened the bottle, she decided to use Meridian Therapy and tap about her rage because she knew she wouldn't be able to sleep unless she could calm down. On a scale of zero to ten, she rated her wrath as one hundred. Within three or four minutes she was completely peaceful. Tapping helped her let go of her outrage, and she decided that she could phone the telephone company the next day and get things resolved. Best of all, she went to bed without drinking and fell asleep immediately.

Doris was also someone who held on to anger. She took offense easily. Sometimes she would go on a shopping spree and act out her anger by "spending at" her boyfriend rather than tell him she was upset with him. Other times she would do underhanded things to get back at those who treated her in ways she thought she didn't deserve.

When Doris began to tap about her anger toward her boyfriend after he criticized her, it brought to mind the many times her mother beat her when she was growing up. Doris was the victim of years of physical abuse. She learned to swallow her rage because if she talked back, she was hurt even more, so she learned to get back at people in other ways.

> As her anger dissipated using Meridian Therapy, Doris worried about releasing her anger. "I don't want to let it go because it helped me survive," she said. With continued tapping Doris realized that she could be free of the anger from the past that was still hurting her and deal with current angers in appropriate ways.

To Vent or Not to Vent

Recent studies show that hitting a punching bag or pounding a pillow doesn't release or reduce the anger. Quite the contrary, acting out the anger tends to lead to more aggressive behavior. Perhaps the old advice to count to ten before you express your anger is good after all. I recommend that you tap your energy points for ten seconds as an even better alternative.

Many men, like Hector, have trouble controlling angry outbursts. Hector developed his own technique: He tapped throughout the day to keep his rage in check. Tapping helped him understand what lay beneath his storminess. Like Doris, he too discovered that he believed he wouldn't be safe without his anger.

Frequently, when tapping, some people discover that sadness, hurt, abandonment, trauma, or fear are waiting to be dealt with. If you are like Hector, start by saying, "Even though I won't be safe if I give up my anger, I profoundly forgive and accept myself." Continue tapping the energy points and notice what comes to mind. It may take a number of rounds to resolve this blocking belief. Only after you feel safe will you be able to tackle the explosive anger problem.

Tap to Improve Relationships

Jason and Eileen fought about everything. They did a lot of yelling, and their fights often escalated to threats of divorce. Once, when he was red-faced with fury and at the end of his patience with Eileen during a counseling session, I asked Jason to tap the energy points while he was seething. After the first round Jason grew a little calmer. As he tapped again, his face softened and tears came to his eyes. "I love her so much," he exclaimed. In that moment Jason realized the depth of his feeling for his wife and forgot what he was upset about.

John Gottman, Ph.D., has been studying couples in his laboratory for more than twenty years. One of his discoveries is that when the heart rate escalates, a person is not able to stay centered. Tapping can "soothe the savage breast." If you are upset with a spouse, child, parent, or friend, rate the intensity of your upset and tap one or two rounds before you begin the conversation. Take the edge off your negative emotion. Then communicate with the other. It works better if you both do it. Couples who bicker and fight may want to use Meridian Therapy as they talk to each other in a narrative style.

Another problem that Dr. Gottman recognized as detrimental to a happy relationship is called "stonewalling." Some people become physiologically overwhelmed or "flooded" when a situation heats up. As a result, they turn off and tune out. It is as if they are paralyzed, unable to say what is going on. Their partner sees this "silent treatment" as a red flag and usually becomes more and more frustrated. The more one partner escalates, trying to get a rise out of the stony partner, the more that partner withdraws. The result can be miserable for both parties.

If you recognize that you or your partner stonewall, use Meridian Therapy to de-escalate the stress as it builds. "Stonewallers" can tap to reduce the reaction to a partner's anger before it overwhelms. The recipients of stonewalling can also tap to keep their reaction from getting out of hand.

Holding On to Your Anger Memories

Linda had a different kind of anger problem. She was an anger collector, still actively upset over happenings of thirty years ago. She lovingly brought out her memories of how others had hurt her over the years and recounted them as if she were sharing a photo album. Linda wasn't sure she wanted to let the past be in the past. Anger was her friend. "It keeps me warm," she explained. Her anger and resentment toward others acted like a shot of adrenaline and made her feel alive. "Anger is the coal that feeds my engine," she said. After Linda decided to heal the past and tapped away the upsetting memories, she felt lighter and more positive.

If you are an anger collector, you can easily get rid of the grudges you have collected using Meridian Therapy. Compile an "Anger List." Make a list of all the people, living or dead, and events from your past and your present that you still feel anger, resentment, frustration, or rage about. You may still hate the kids in the fourth grade who didn't pick you for their team.

Be specific and concrete. Rather than write "Mother" as a topic, list many memories that still make you angry with your mother, as if you are writing the Table of Contents for your autobiography. "My third birthday party," "She wanted a girl and had me instead," "When she sent me away to school," or, "She bought me ugly shoes and everyone made fun of me." The list doesn't have to be in chronological order. Make each entry brief. Don't expect to complete the Anger List in one sitting. As the days and weeks go by, other memories will come to mind that you can add to your list.

When you are ready, set aside some time to eradicate old wounds. Start anywhere on your Anger List. Pick whatever topic appeals to you. Name the experience you feel angry about and use the Five Simple Steps. The irritation may dissolve in a few seconds for some of the memories. Others will take longer to dissipate. Getting rid of old angers doesn't mean that you will no longer feel any angry feelings. Events that you don't like will continue to occur in your life. Keep current. Don't let angry sludge clog up your life. Tap it away as soon as you feel it.

To Forgive Is Divine

You may wonder how it is possible to forgive a rapist or thief. It isn't easy. After Kurt tapped about his rage toward his physically abusive father, he felt sadness and compassion, but he couldn't forgive his father for all the pain he had inflicted on Kurt for so many years.

Finally Kurt realized that holding on to his anger was causing him unwanted stress. Kurt created a new affirmation. As he tapped he said, "My happiness and well-being are no longer dependent on my father's apology." He felt as if a heavy weight lifted from his chest. Other affirmations you may want to use are: "I forgive you. I know that you were doing the best you could." Or "I forgive you. You were a prisoner of your own history."

Her father, grandfather, and brother had molested Sunny as a child. She was angry with God for letting that happen to her. When Meridian Therapy healed the past traumas, she was able to forgive by tapping and saying, "I forgive you, God. I know that was the way things needed to be."

Anxiety Can Help or Hurt

If early man hadn't felt fear in the face of danger, we wouldn't be here today. Anxiety, the reaction to fear, is a basic survival skill. We experience it every day. You may get butterflies in your stomach before you have to make a presentation, become tense when your spouse criticizes you, or feel your heart race when you think you are in danger. Worry and tension are the hallmarks of anxiety. Today you are not in danger of being eaten by an angry tiger, but many of us fear carjackers or gunmen who heedlessly fire into crowds at schools, at post offices, and in the workplace. We are concerned for our safety and our loved ones' protection.

Emily, mother of three, suffered from anticipation anxiety. She was extremely worried about a trip her six-year-old daughter Sally was going to take during summer vacation. Sally was going with her aunt to visit relatives far away. Emily recalled that she had a terrible fear of her mother leaving her when she was small. Emily cried at kindergarten and wouldn't let mother drop her off at birthday parties. As she tapped about her fear over Sally's trip she said, "I couldn't live if something happened to her. She is so special. I always wanted a girl. First I had two boys and thought I'd never have what I wanted so much. I don't deserve it."

Emily's anxiety was related to a mixture of her own childhood fears and her negative core belief that she was unworthy. Emily kept tapping about her unworthiness and worry and was able to reduce her anxiety. Later Sally went on vacation and had a grand time. She arrived back home safe and sound and was met by her relaxed mother.

Worries can turn into solutions with Meridian Therapy. Rachel's daughter was graduating from medical school and had invited a number of family members to attend. One was Rachel's sister Mollie. Rachel and Mollie had had a falling out and weren't speaking to each other. Rachel was tense. There would be a celebration after the graduation, and she was worried about having an anxiety attack when she saw Mollie. Rachel began to tap about her worry. As her distress disappeared, she decided to phone her sister and talk to her, perhaps heal the rift between them. The call was a success and the graduation was a joyous affair for all.

Meridian Therapy can help you get rid of momentary anxiety swiftly. Jake found himself wide awake at two in the morning. A nightmare left him distressed and frightened. Fortunately he remembered to use Meridian Therapy and went back to sleep in a few minutes. Another surprised person was Hal. An hour into gum surgery, Hal began to feel anxious when he heard an ominous scraping sound. Since he was immobilized by a large protective bib and unable to use his hands to tap, he began to imagine stimulating the energy points. After three imaginary rounds, he was calm once more.

There Is a Name for It

When worry becomes excessive and you have difficulty controlling it, you may be suffering from GAD, Generalized

Anxiety Disorder. GAD is more than everyday worry. In addition to tension, you may also feel restless or on edge, have trouble concentrating, feel irritable or tired, have trouble falling asleep, or have your muscles feel tense. The Anxiety Disorders Association of America claims that four million people endure this problem. If your anxiety has reached a point where it is interfering with your life, continue to use Meridian Therapy and consult your doctor or a mental health professional.

An Rx for Guilt

There is no medication for guilt. Guilt comes from not living up to what you think others expect of you. Guilt is instilled in us from early childhood when there are many "no-no's" to deal with. We are made to feel inadequate or shamed when we don't follow the rules of right and wrong. Guilt dissolves quickly with a few rounds of Meridian Therapy.

Before the advent of Meridian Therapy it might have taken years of psychotherapy for a person to come to terms with long-standing guilt or shame. Ira was haunted by forty-five years of guilt because he felt responsible for an accident that killed a playmate, since he had encouraged his friend to go on an outing where the accident took place. Since then Ira had been unable to cry. The long-term guilt kept him from leading a satisfying life. He avoided forming meaningful relationships with people and even kept distant from his family.

At first Ira was afraid to approach the memory because it was too painful. He began to work with a therapist trained in Meridian Therapy. With her guidance, Ira tapped about his responsibility for the tragedy and his guilt. He felt more relaxed and less burdened. With Meridian Therapy he didn't have to relive the trauma of the accident in order to heal it. In about an hour he was able to accept in his heart that he was just a child at the time of the accident and was doing the best he could. What a major breakthrough after a lifetime of hell! The guilt was gone. Later he remarked, "Now it's behind me. I don't think about it anymore."

Soraya couldn't forgive herself for a comment she had made to a friend five years ago. The relationship was never the same after that. Soraya felt a constant "hum of guilt" in her head that kept her from being all she could be. She wasn't able to release the guilt until she healed her belief that "I don't deserve to get over this guilt." In less than a half-hour Soraya was able to forgive herself and decided to make amends to the person she had harmed. She felt a renewed energy in her life. "I feel energized and alive in a way that I haven't experienced for too many years to count. I am now fully alive," she rejoiced.

Guilt or Shame?

We often use the words *guilt* and *shame* interchangeably. They are not the same. Guilt means "I did something wrong." Shame means "I am something wrong." Shame implies that you are basically bad through and through, flawed, unacceptable. Shame can permeate your life and block you from succeeding. Start by applying the Meridian Therapy technique for the feeling of shame. When you know that you are not basically bad, you will regain the power to improve your life.

To eliminate guilty feelings, you may want to start by tapping as you say, "Even though I don't deserve to be free of this guilt or shame, I love and accept myself." After you have transformed this belief, you can tap about "this guilt" or tap about the physical sensation in the body where guilt is buried. Sometimes it is in the throat where you can't express your emotions; often it can be in the stomach or heart. The variation of Meridian Therapy called "The Body Knows," in Chapter 3, shows you how to follow the discomfort throughout the body. To process a specific memory that is the origin of your guilt or shame, use the Five Simple Steps or the "See a Movie in Your Head" technique on page 192.

It is important to tap until you can forgive yourself for whatever you think you did or said that has kept you guilt-ridden. Kristen, who, as a child had been raped by a neighbor, felt intense shame about being molested. On some level she blamed herself for what happened. This is common among people sexually molested or physically abused in childhood. As adults they still believe they were to blame. They often think, "I should have known better." When you use Meridian Therapy, you will be able to see the past from a new vantage point and put it to rest.

Relief from Grief and Loss

Grief, sadness, and love-loss can also be remedied with Meridian Therapy. The death of a loved one is one of the most painful things we can experience. The grieving process is a natural one and can take time. Some people cannot stop grieving for many years. Yet the pain can be relieved. Leah, Rita, and Corinne dealt with different kinds of loss.

Leah lost her husband after fifty years of marriage. She was lonely, sad, depressed, and angry, and wasn't sleeping. She tapped about her sadness and inability to sleep and was soon able to have restful nights. The most difficult time for her was being alone at night. She began to sit with her husband's picture and tap while feeling the grief without words. It eased the pain. As time went on, she needed to do it less often to relax and calm herself.

Rita was inconsolable. She and Herb had set a wedding date, but he called it off and ended the relationship. Love-loss was devastating her life. As the day of the wedding neared, she began to feel even more upset thinking about what she would never have. Rita decided to deal with her problem by going to the chapel and performing a private ritual surrounded by the decorative flowers and candles. She thought it would help to assuage her grief.

A few days before her visit to the chapel I helped her deal with her feelings about being jilted using Meridian Therapy. Later she reported, "I went to church and saw the flowers and candles, but I only stayed a short while. I told myself, enough is enough! Now I think that maybe there could be someone better for me."

Corinne used Meridian Therapy to take the edge off her grief. Her teenage son had been killed in a gang fight five years before, yet her grief was as painful as if it had just happened. Every day was filled with reminders of him that brought tears. She paid frequent visits to his grave. After just a few minutes of tapping Corinne felt significant relief. She stopped feeling the constant pain. Her life was no longer built around the wound of her loss, and she was able to keep his memory in her heart as she went on with her life.

Be Gentle with Yourself

There are no limiting rules for using Meridian Therapy to heal grief. Some people will benefit from tapping while they cry. Others will find that tapping as they remember certain moments will be most helpful. Leah tapped as she silently felt the emotions of loneliness, anger, and depression after her husband's death. Help yourself in whatever way you think works best. Just a few moments of tapping your energy points will be worthwhile.

How to Tell If You Are Clinically Depressed

Losing someone or something precious usually leads to depression. Even the loss of a pet can catapult a person into despair. Extreme stress is also a factor in creating depression. "Downsizing" has caused many people to go into a decline. As many as 20 percent of women and 10 percent of men will suffer an episode of clinical depression at some time in their lives.

We all have days when we feel down in the dumps or blue. However, there is a difference between the normal ups and downs of life and clinical depression. Clinical depression can be mild or severe, but either way you feel weighed down by things and generally believe it will never get better. Clinical depression often affects your appetite, and you may either overeat or lose your desire for food. The same happens with sleep. You may have trouble sleeping or have trouble staying awake. There is no joy in living. Things you used to look forward to seem uninteresting, and you don't have the energy to do them.

If you find that your low mood is keeping you from working or taking care of yourself and you feel so worthless you are thinking of killing yourself, you must see a doctor. Today there are many effective ways to deal with depression. You may decide to use antidepressants, alternative medications or herbs, counseling, or a combination of these. First check it out with a specialist.

Keep Tapping to Improve Your Mood

Even if you are already under care for depression, Meridian Therapy will assist you in lightening your mood and moving out of the doldrums. Tapping can help you feel better, but depression will not disappear overnight. Brent was taking medication but was still extremely down. He began to tap for his depression twice a day, when he woke up and at bedtime. After six weeks he felt so good, he was able to stop his twice-a-day regime. Make Meridian Therapy your friend to deal with depression. Tap as often as possible every day.

On days I wake up disgruntled and downhearted I look forward to practicing my Daily Meridian Therapy Workout. Sometimes I know what is making me gloomy, other times I don't. Spending ten minutes to release my unhappiness always gets results. My mood lifts so I can go on with my day, and often my feeling of depression totally disappears and is replaced with a positive state of mind.

Life is like the seasons. We have emotional summers, autumns, winters and springs. At times we can go through many feelings in one day. We all feel stress, anger, anxiety, guilt, shame, sadness, and depression at some time. Now that you know relief is at your fingertips, you can take the edge off intense negative emotions and tap your way into the sunshine of happy thoughts.

chapter five

Be the Best You Can Be: End Performance Anxiety

We have all experienced the fear of looking foolish in front of others at some time in our lives. Performance anxiety is a major problem in our society where the number-one fear is the fear of public speaking. The majority of performers, actors, dancers, musicians, and sports stars experience stage fright. Salespeople worry about failing to close sales. Lovers often hesitate in the privacy of the bedroom because they tell themselves they will disappoint their partner when it comes to sexual performance. Students dread exams, writing papers, and giving reports, fearing poor grades. Let's look at some of these fears affecting millions everywhere. I will show how you can eliminate performance anxiety forever.

In Front of All Those People!

Rose, the curriculum programmer at a college where I was teaching classes, exclaimed, "I don't know how you can get up in front of all those people all the time!" She was imagining how it would be for herself and cringed at the thought. She preferred her own job where she only had to converse with people one on one. The idea of so many eyes looking at her filled her with terror.

Dennis experienced a different symptom. When he had to speak in front of more than three people his voice would change. It became constricted and whispery, as if something were choking him.

David had a strong fear of speaking in public or teaching a group. Tapping eliminated his fear in a half-hour. Six months later David was asked to conduct a training session for forty people. He was worried that his victory over fear of public speaking wouldn't last. Here's what happened when he tested the fear.

> Attendees began to arrive. Instead of feeling as if I was walking the plank, I enjoyed meeting them. I still believed that the problems would come when I was introduced, and when I actually had to do something. To my enormous surprise and delight nothing bad happened! Even better, I was totally relaxed. My pulse didn't rise one extra beat. My voice was firm, breathing OK, mind clear and receptive. What a feeling!

Eliminate Your Fear Now!

You can help yourself right now to overcome the fear of speaking in front of large or small groups. Begin by thinking about your fear. Clarify what terrifies you. Do you relate to any of these fear thoughts?

- I am worried about being unprepared.
- I will forget what I want to say in the middle of my talk.
- I will lose my voice.
- They will laugh at me.
- All those eyes will be on me.
- I will be judged and found wanting.
- I will freeze when answering questions from the audience.

Tap the fear thought that worries you. Become aware of thoughts, beliefs, or memories that come to mind. Treat each one separately until you feel free of every concern. This is how David overcame his fear, and so did Johanna.

When Johanna was invited to give a talk in her hometown she was both elated and terrified. She was especially fearful of having all those eyes on her, judging her. I asked her who exactly was judging her. She immediately named a group of people who were friends of her parents, people who had watched her grow up. As soon as Johanna knew whom "those eyes" belonged to she visualized them as she tapped. Shortly, she realized that they would be there to honor her, not to criticize her.

Heal Past Embarrassment

Create a video in your head recalling a time you felt embarrassed before a group. Early unhappy experiences often linger for years. Some of us shudder to remember flubbing a word in a spelling bee or class play in elementary school. Go to the worst part of the memory. Did your teacher criticize you in public? Did others laugh at you? Rate your discomfort as you employ the Five Simple Steps procedure. Continue until you no longer react when you reminisce. As you process the early memory, other humiliating moments may come to mind. Use Meridian Therapy on any that still sting.

Mentally create a positive outcome for a public appearance coming up. Imagine a new video of your worst-case scenario. Start with the moment you were asked to make the presentation. Go through each step of the experience as you think it will unfold. Begin with the earliest moment you usually feel fearful—the night before, driving to the location, or waiting to be introduced. Stop yourself as soon as you experience anxiety or fear. Tap until there is no negative emotional charge.

Go back to your script. Start again, going past the part you have just treated to imagine what follows. Stop at the next sign of upset and treat that until you feel neutral. Keep this up until you can run through the entire projected experience, seeing yourself performing with ease and enjoying it.

Don't Wait to Feel Good

Often people want me to treat them a few days before a frightening event. They don't realize they can avoid enduring weeks of anxiety if they eliminate the fear as soon as they are aware of it. Address the fear immediately, and you won't have to use Meridian Therapy over and over again, because the fear will not come back. If necessary, tap before the event whenever you feel nervous thinking about it. It is OK to tap during a break or intermission if anxiety mounts.

Improve Sports Performance

Better performance is the goal of all athletes. Sports are an area in which Meridian Therapy can ease the pressure of competition and striving for excellence that create intense stress. In gymnastics, diving, golf, bowling, or tennis the focus is on the individual. Team sports provoke anxiety too. The tension builds on Little League or children's soccer fields as well as in professional arenas. We spend a great deal of time rooting for our favorites and putting even more pressure on those who are already outstanding to outdo themselves.

Meridian Therapy can be helpful in any sport. You already know that part of every game is mental. Negative beliefs can cause discomfort and tension in your body. Meridian Therapy eliminates the mental roadblocks to success and creates a feeling of relaxation that will help you concentrate on improving your skills. Tap to diminish stress before a practice or a game. Concentrate on physical sensations—tension in your body, butterflies in your stomach, or any aches and pains.

Do you spend more time than you want agonizing about your performance? Do you push yourself to do better and worry about what others think, whether you are playing a friendly game or a competitive tournament? Tap to eliminate these sabotaging states.

- Scare thoughts ("I'm not going to make this shot"; "I'm having an off day")
- Worries about your "form"
- Anxiety about competing
- Comparing yourself to others

- Fear of getting a bad score
- Fear of losing

Thousands of people have significantly improved their performance and their scores by using power therapies like Meridian Therapy.

A Good Golfer Gets Better

I went out to the driving range with my husband's coworker Andrew to demonstrate the advantages of Meridian Therapy for golf. I asked him to use twelve balls, hitting four balls with three different clubs. After each shot he was to rate the result as "not good," "pretty good," or "very good." Andrew is a passionate golfer who plays frequently. Most of his ratings were "very good." I began to wonder how Meridian Therapy could improve his already outstanding ability.

After Andrew hit all twelve balls, I asked him to practice Meridian Therapy while thinking about any stress he might be feeling. He realized that he was still worried about a difficult situation at work that morning. After tapping about that problem and worries about his swing, Andrew took twelve more balls and repeated the experiment. This time he tapped before each swing. Since Andrew was already a fine golfer, I thought that maybe he would just hit more "very good" shots than in the previous twelve tries.

Instead we were both surprised and delighted that Andrew began to hit balls that he rated not as "very good" but "perfect!" He excitedly reported that he hit three balls in the exact same spot, one after another. Andrew has continued to use Meridian Therapy to help with his game.

Get Rid of Your Mental Baggage

When you are using Meridian Therapy for sports performance, take stock of anything that could contribute to stress. Tension will take away from the quality of your game. Ask yourself, "Is anything on my mind that is worrying me about work, family, money, health, the state of the world?" Some people use sports to relieve the pressures of the day but can't shake negative thoughts or feelings of the past few hours even while playing. You can tap away the unneeded negatives before you get to the golf course, basketball court, football field, or baseball diamond. Tap them before you begin to play.

Pitcher of the Year

Pat Ahearne was named Pitcher of the Year in the Australian Baseball League. Pat believes that "the difference between the average athlete and the elite player is much more mental than physical." Pat tapped to eliminate the mental and emotional barriers preventing him from consistently producing excellent games.

His statistics the season before and the season after treatment:

Hits given up: Before, 43; After, 15
Earned runs: Before, 17; After, 4
Walks given up: Before, 18; After, 7
Earned run average: Before, 3.33; After, 0.87

You Are Never Too Young to Tap

You don't have to be a professional player to benefit from tapping. Meridian Therapy is a great way to help young players. Rhonda, mother of two ball-playing sons, noticed that her seven-year-old had trouble catching the ball because he was afraid of being hit by it. His older brother taught him how to tap, and in just a few minutes he was catching the ball. Both boys also use Meridian Therapy during games to keep their spirits up when their teams are losing.

Undo Self-Sabotage

Keeping our spirits up takes effort when there is pressure to excel. We frequently hold ourselves under a microscope, looking for all the things we do wrong rather than congratulating ourselves on what we do right. Many golfers, baseball players, gymnasts, skaters, and tennis players have an immediate negative self-criticism after each swing, serve, or move. The moment you focus on what you did wrong and hear yourself thinking critically, tap the negative statement. What about your score bothers you? Although you want to be a better player, tapping to eliminate how you pressure yourself to score well may remove extra tension, actually allowing you to do well and enjoy yourself more.

Underlying self-doubt can create barriers to success. You may not even be aware you have a mindset that says, "I'm a failure," I'm not good enough," or, "I don't deserve to win." If you are tapping regularly and are still getting poor results, study Chapter 13, "Beliefs That Block Success." If you think you'll never make the "A" team, your negative view of yourself may be affecting many areas of your life, not just sports.

Aches and Pains Go Away

"No pain, no gain" is taught to many young athletes. A soccer mom used tapping to help some of her child's teammates with their aches and pains before the game. For the affirmation she suggested they say, "Even though I have this pain, I will play my best game." The players discovered that their pains went away and they played better. Teams can tap before a game and between periods, innings, or halves. Players may choose to target their specific shortcomings or the problem of losing focus. Meridian Therapy can be fine-tuned for whatever a player needs.

Gymnasts and skaters face the risk of injury when there is pressure to do even more intricate and difficult movements. A teenaged gymnast told me that sometimes she hesitates before doing a difficult move but doesn't know what stops her. I urged her to tap while experiencing the sensation in her gut that makes her stop herself, rather than try to figure it out in her head. Using Meridian Therapy, you don't have to know why in order for change to take place. She stopped balking after tapping away the scary feeling.

Fear of Injury—Past, Present, and Future

A common problem for many athletes is the fear of injury or memory of severe injury. Becky felt nervous when she had to work on the balance beam during gymnastics practice. She had recently healed from a sprained ankle suffered when she fell, and every time she got on the beam she remembered the pain. She rated her anxiety at number eight and tapped. She tapped the memory of the fall, the fear, and the pain until remembering no longer affected her. She was able to compete fearlessly after that and scored higher in competitions.

After you have been hurt, you may also develop a fear you will be injured again the next time you compete. When you are being held back in your performance because of an old trauma, think about your worst injury or your most recent injury and follow the Five Simple Steps until the memory is neutralized, as Becky did. If you are obsessed about the future, pinpoint the thought that generates fear: "I will sprain my wrist when I land," "I will cut my foot," "I will hurt my head," "I will straddle the balance beam." Tap about the event you are projecting will happen until you feel free of the fear.

Don't wait until you are at the playing field to work on your performance. Tap before you leave home. Tap in the locker room. Practice Meridian Therapy on the putting green or driving range or at the batting cage.

Musical Performance

Meridian Therapy can benefit musicians in two important ways. First, relaxing tensions can enhance performance skills. Second, anxieties about playing in front of an audience can be eliminated.

Alan Handelsman is a therapist and musician. He works with aspiring flute, saxophone, and clarinet players from age five to adult. According to Alan:

One of the most powerful ways to immediately enhance performance is to release inhibitions of breath. I have the student play a selection. Then I have him rate how much air he's getting in. We do one or two rounds of tapping and then rate the breath again. Usually the rating goes from a seven or eight to a nine or ten. Then the student repeats the same piece. Without exception, he plays better. The tone will be better. Instrument response is faster and easier. Usually the student plays faster with no realization that he is. Often he reports being less concerned with making mistakes.

Students will want to tap when they are frustrated while learning a new piece that seems hard or if they don't want to practice. All musicians can use Meridian Therapy to improve concentration, ease of playing and touch, and to avoid making the same mistake over and over again. Fear of making a mistake or harsh self-criticism will also ease.

Facing the Audience

Performance can be scary for even the most proficient musician. Getting up in front of an audience often creates high anxiety. Hold your instrument and tap while getting in touch with your general feeling of nervousness. Concentrate on the part of the experience that scares you the most. It helps to think about the presentation as if you were watching yourself on film. Start with the day of the performance and, step by step, run through the entire day, noting when the tension arises. Stop at each upsetting moment and tap the stress away. You may find that you are most disturbed before the performance or only when you are on the stage. Some people are terrified they will forget the notes or make a mistake. Others are worried about the audience reaction and judgment of their playing. Meridian Therapy will allay stage fright. However, if you think you need to, continue to tap before going on stage or during intermission.

When memories of past unpleasant experiences or poor performances come to mind, use Meridian Therapy for each memory. Pay attention to all the elements that trouble you. When you have reduced each one to zero, go back over the entire sequence from the beginning to make sure you have treated all the parts. Singers, dancers, and actors have many of the same anxieties as musicians. They can follow the same steps to improve performance and remove the barriers to success.

Sexual Performance Fears

Despite what magazines say about everyone having hotter sex than you do, apparently it isn't true. A study led by University of Chicago researchers revealed that more than 40 percent of American women aged eighteen to fifty-nine, and nearly a third of men, report some kind of sexual problem. The most common complaints of those studied were lack of interest, loss of desire or enjoyment, performance anxiety, and inability to achieve or delay orgasm.

Fear of rejection by a loved one causes many men and women to sit home alone. Worries about attractiveness and the ability to be a good lover may hamper your love life. Sexual performance can be a lifelong stress. Women worry about having orgasms. Men worry about maintaining erections and pleasing their partners. Both sexes worry about looking good and "winning" a mate.

Breakthroughs in the Bedroom

Jack and Barbara admitted to their therapist that they hadn't had sex in over a year. They were reluctant to pursue the matter. However, they were willing to tap about their fear of talking about sex. They each released that fear in a few rounds, but they still weren't willing to continue the discussion. That was the only time they addressed their problem, yet when they went on vacation a month later they renewed their sexual relationship and had a wonderful time.

Kelly's marriage suffered because of her disgust about semen. She was revolted by the thought of having semen on her skin or near her face. Any kind of oral sex was out of bounds. Meridian Therapy eliminated her fear and enabled her to be more sexually free with her husband than she had ever been in the five years they had been married. She felt relaxed and less inhibited. Kelly was able to ask her husband to touch her in ways that excited her and stopped holding back from pleasuring her husband.

Patsy and Jeff decided to use Meridian Therapy in the bedroom to remove the resistant thoughts that interfered with the moment of pleasure and kept them from enjoying sex fully. Some of Patsy's negative thoughts were: "Other women can, but not me." "Is he bored?" and "Will I disappoint him?" Patsy released the concerns and fears that were blocking her enjoyment and self-confidence during sex by using Mental Tapping. She was able to return immediately to the excitement of the moment. Jeff too released stress-producing ideas. Patsy and Jeff's lovemaking breakthrough resulted in mutual multiple and sustained orgasms.

The most important sexual organ is the brain. As Patsy and Jeff discovered, sexual satisfaction and enjoyment are strongly influenced by your thoughts and beliefs. When you think of failure or tell yourself you aren't capable, lovable, or expert in bed, you take yourself away from the intimacy of the moment. According to Patsy, "Every time my thoughts would wander from focus on pleasure to other concerns, I would release them by imagining tapping the energy points, returning my mind to center. The result was that it turned lovemaking into a meditation."

Coming Down from the Bleachers

In a classic Woody Allen movie there is a bedroom scene in which Woody is making love to his leading lady, yet, at the same time, he is sitting in the bleachers, watching himself and making derogatory observations. That is called "spectatoring" and is a common hazard to any kind of performance success. When you watch yourself, you can't be totally in the moment, nor can you be totally one with your partner and your pleasure.

The worst part of "spectatoring" is that it is inherently negative. When you see yourself from outside yourself, you are usually criticizing your every move and every word. You may also be telling yourself that you are letting your partner down. Many people report thinking they are ugly, fat, wrinkled, old, anything but sexy and desirable. Tap to transform critical thoughts about your body or your technique.

Meridian Therapy has allowed men and women to overcome aversion to kissing, sex without passion, boredom with one's partner, inability to reach orgasm, and other problems of desire. Fear, guilt, or anxiety may hinder your happiness. A strict religious upbringing may have instilled shame about sex and kept you from feeling comfortable with your partner. Meridian Therapy can extinguish this kind of shame. Tap in private or, better yet, tap with your partner as you share your fears or worries about being desirable or successful. You have nothing to lose and a great deal of pleasure to gain.

Overcoming Fear of Rejection

Fear of rejection influences how you behave, what you do, and what you don't do. A wise man said, "If you think you can or you think you can't, you're right." No one likes to be told "No." Do you avoid situations in which you might experience rejection? Some people seem to have tough skins, yet you find yourself falling apart at the least sign of being turned down.

Negative beliefs can cause you to stop yourself before you even start. The most common thoughts that block success are about not deserving to have success, love, approval, or prosperity, or fear of being harmed in some way if you succeed. Harboring these thoughts leads to feeling unworthy, unlovable, or powerless. Despite your best attempts to succeed, the secret conviction that you deserve to fail thwarts every effort.

The Power of No

Salespeople aren't the only ones who try to avoid being turned down. We all risk rejection when we interview for a job, apply to enter college or graduate school, ask someone for a date, or propose marriage. Many writers and artists

Life or Death of a Salesman

Ken's main fear as a salesman was making cold calls. He just couldn't get started phoning. He would putter around the house and find all kinds of excuses not to pick up the threatening instrument. He eliminated the fear in a brief session of Meridian Therapy with me. Ken hadn't uncovered the reasons behind his procrastination, but the dread disappeared as he tapped. It hasn't returned.

Sales fears include being reluctant to approach wealthy people, authoritative people, or total strangers. Even if you have the gift of gab you may be hampered by other secret undermining thoughts.

never try to sell their pieces because they believe they will be devastated by rejection.

Your first experience may have been in childhood when you weren't chosen for a team. Maybe you decided you aren't appealing when you weren't invited to someone's birthday party or didn't receive a valentine in elementary school. Asking someone on a date can be excruciating for a shy person. If early memories still plague you, use Meridian Therapy to put them successfully to rest.

Danny and Janine had been friends for some time. Now he wanted to have more than a friendship with her but feared losing her entirely if he let his feelings be known. Danny used Meridian Therapy to overcome his nervousness about talking to her. Although rejection can cause heartache, he now felt strong and confident about taking the risk. He talked to her about his romantic feelings. The bad news was that Janine wanted to just remain friends. The good news was that thanks to Meridian Therapy, Danny still felt good about himself after he had been rebuffed.

Chances of being rejected are present all through our lives. Getting a job, keeping a job, asking for a raise, and competing for a promotion, are part of life. Running for office in your class, club, or government is risky, because only one will win. It may not always be you. Are you willing to take that chance? You can use Meridian Therapy to get yourself ready to take risks as well as deal with the aftereffects if you are rejected.

Prepare for a confrontation in advance. Tap as soon as you think about a situation you feel nervous about. Listen to each self-defeating thought that is whispering in your mind. Zap it as you tap it! You can practice Meridian Therapy on your way to a meeting if you are anxious. Instead of berating yourself when you are rejected, naming yourself a failure, use Narrative Meridian Therapy to think about what happened. As you eliminate feelings of despair and self-criticism, you will think up new solutions.

Achieving Financial Success

What is your definition of money? Here is what happened when I asked Connie and Stuart that question. Connie and Stuart, a couple in their sixties, were stuck in gridlock because of their beliefs about money. Connie was extremely anxious about spending and saving. She excitedly told me, "Money is something you have to save up so you'll have it for a rainy day." Stuart was irate. "Money is something you use to make more money with," he explained. "Money is a tool."

Connie saw money as something limited and finite, while Stuart thought of money as a fluid medium that was flexible and growing. As she tapped, Connie was able to acknowledge that Stuart had been very successful in business using money as a tool, and Stuart came to understand Connie's fears about being widowed and unable to take care of herself. They were then able to resume their loving relationship.

What Do You Believe?

Is money a medium of exchange for goods and services, a doorway to freedom, something always out of your grasp, a burden, or an abstract idea? I once asked a group to complete this sentence: Rich people _____. Some of the answers were rather surprising: Rich people are mean. Rich people take advantage of others. Rich people inherit their money. Rich people are insensitive to others. Conversely, these people answered, "Poor people are the salt of the earth," and "Poor people get into heaven." No wonder they were having trouble increasing their prosperity!

If you are struggling with this problem, think about your family's attitude toward money and success. What kind of role models did you have? Did your family disparage money or enjoy wealth? Did they tell you that you could or would succeed? Did they say one thing but do another? List all the negative beliefs your role models taught you were the truth about money and about your prosperity. Ask yourself if you still want to live by them. Here are a few examples to consider:

- Money is the root of all evil.
- Money is a burden. People will try to rip me off.
- Women can't earn as much as men.

- Women are supposed to be taken care of.
- If I become rich I will forget my friends and family.
- If I become rich, my friends won't like me anymore.
- I shouldn't do better than my father/mother.
- People who have a lot of money have gotten it in illegal ways.
- Saving money is hoarding and it's wrong to hoard money.
- I can amass money, but I can't hold on to it.
- Spiritual people should not have a lot of money.
- I deserve to suffer. I deserve to be poor.
- Nothing ever works for me. I never get a break in life.

When his homeowner's insurance, car insurance, and income tax were all due at the same time Phil became overwhelmed. His anxiety kept him from figuring out how to make ends meet. He believed that he never got breaks, and that financial troubles would stalk him forever. Tapping helped him break the cycle of fear thoughts. Once he was calm he was able to figure out a way to meet his obligations. He discovered that he would have enough money to pay his bills if he cut back on some of his other activities for a while.

Words from the Wise

A wise minister I once knew said, "The Truth with a capital T is true for everyone, everywhere, all the time. If it isn't, then it's just your opinion, and you can change your opinion." If your beliefs are hurting you more than helping you, perhaps they are only opinions. Use Meridian Therapy to target each idea that stops you from enjoying financial success.

Too Scared to Score Well

Opinions about our self-worth and capabilities begin in childhood. School brings pressure to score well on tests and compete with peers. At any age, test-taking anxiety can be paralyzing. Your brain feels like it's filled with cotton. The answers that were there the night before have vanished. As you mature, you may be faced with important entrance exams or license exams. The most common is the SAT that many high-school students sit for. Later, exams to enter graduate school or professional training in medical or law school may create enormous anticipatory anxiety. Some people have failed the bar or license exams two or three times. Others have trouble renewing their driver's license.

Farrah's mother brought her to see me because although she is a very bright girl and excellent student, her test scores weren't reflecting her abilities. It was final exams week, an excellent time to test the efficacy of Meridian Therapy. I asked Farrah to tell me what she experienced when she was taking a test. "I feel nervous and shaky. I am scared I won't remember what I just studied. It's like my brain is turned off."

Next I asked her to tell me how anxious she felt just talking about the coming exams. Her anxiety was very high. We tapped about the overall problem of taking tests and then on each of her negative thoughts and doubts. Some worries took a few minutes for the discomfort to reach zero. Others took only seconds.

Finally, I asked Farrah to picture herself at the test she was going to take the very next day. "Be aware of any signs of stress or new negative thoughts," I said. There were one or two that we quickly treated. Before the hour was over Farrah was calm and confident. She did much better on her finals than ever before.

Forever Grad School

Eleanor, a graduate student, was terribly upset and fearful. She was stuck in the midst of writing her doctoral dissertation. Time was running out. Her professors were pressuring her to finish. She had extended her training so long that she was out of money and very far from her home in France. Eleanor was so stressed she couldn't think straight. Without a Ph.D., she would never realize her career dreams.

Anger and fear were keeping Eleanor stuck. She felt angry because her advisor was pushing her to slant her paper in a way that went against all that Eleanor believed in. She felt powerless and enraged. If she refused, her career would be ruined. If she gave in and wrote a paper to please her professor, she was going against all her values and betraying herself. How could she stay in her advisor's good graces and be true to herself? He could harm her chances of advancement if she went against his wishes. No wonder she was stuck!

Eleanor used Meridian Therapy to take the edge off her stress so she could think clearly. She soon came up with some solutions and strategies for handling her nemesis diplomatically. Tapping about her situation and her values strengthened her self-esteem. She discovered a way to write her paper that both pleased her professor and was true to her own knowledge of her field. As she felt better about herself, she felt less in awe of him. She began to write with ease and finished her dissertation before the deadline.

Facing the Orals

Meridian Therapy enabled Paul to achieve an important goal. He had to pass an oral exam to become a licensed psychotherapist. He had some doubts about how well he knew the subject matter, but the main component of his anxiety was the worry that the examiners wouldn't like him, might think he was stupid, or were going to be mean to him. As he tapped he was able to understand that his negative beliefs were mainly fantasies. He soon felt more and more confident about taking the test and reminded himself that if he felt stressed at the exam site, he could use Meridian Therapy in the waiting room before he was called. He went to the oral exam in a relaxed state and passed confidently.

Advice for Parents

Fears about schoolwork and performance begin as soon as we enter school. You can't start using Meridian Therapy early enough. It doesn't matter if your child is in the first grade and worried about a spelling test, in junior high worried about giving a report in front of the class, or in high school preparing for the SATs.

Meridian Therapy can help your children with many of their school problems with a little help from you. If the child is quite young, you can gently tap the child's energy points while speaking about her unhappy feelings like this: "Sarah is feeling very sad. She missed five words on her spelling test. She feels awful." Talk about the trouble and tap until the child is over her unhappiness. Let her decide what to do about her difficulty with spelling. Because parents are so strongly bonded with their offspring, it is sometimes easier for them to tap as a surrogate while talking for the child. The result is the same. The child will begin to feel better.

Target the difficulty. If a child is scared to take a test the next day, have him think about it, experience the fear, and tap. Fear of not remembering what was studied and fear of getting a poor grade or failing may create distress. Tapping will

---

Attitude Matters

If you are working with your child, listen for disparaging self-talk. This is what happened when Frank tried to assist his daughter.

I was helping my daughter with her math homework. She was having difficulty understanding and was close to tears, saying, "I'm useless at this, I will never understand it." I was getting a bit frustrated since I had explained it every way I could, and she still didn't get it. Then the lightbulb went off in my head and I told her to tap as she said, "Even though I can't understand this stuff..." After two rounds of tapping, with me tapping along with her, we were both able to continue. She immediately grasped the concept we had been struggling with and completed her homework easily. What's most wonderful is that she has reversed her feelings about her inadequacy with math.

---

remove the dread of exams and promote calm. Tapping during a test to quiet anxiety is not considered cheating. However, it won't improve the results if a student hasn't studied.

Ready, Set, Go!

The large and small events that trouble you in your daily life can be dealt with in a short time when you use Meridian Therapy. Once you get used to realizing that a few taps will reduce your worries and doubts, performance anxieties can become a thing of the past.

chapter six

How to Be Free from Fear Forever

Meridian Therapy dispels fear quickly and permanently. Whether you have a momentary fright or a long-standing dread, you will realize dramatic results through tapping your meridian points. The most wonderful benefit is that the fear leaves effortlessly. It is as if it never existed. You may even forget how terrified you used to be, like Ann, who was afraid of driving a curvy stretch of road near her home. After tapping rapidly eliminated her fear, she drove without noticing the curves.

Fear or Phobia?

Many people label themselves phobic because they have had fear for a long time. There is a difference between fear and phobia. A fear is an unpleasant emotion caused by the awareness or anticipation of danger. You may be afraid of driving on the freeway in the fog because you can't see the car in front of you and conjure up the possibility of a collision. You may fear going to the dentist because it might be painful. Getting put in a closet as a punishment or prank can lead to a lifelong fear of enclosed spaces like elevators. Many people are afraid of dogs, cats, or insects because they were once hurt or scared by them. No matter the origin of the fear, you can easily and quickly eliminate it with Meridian Therapy, just as many others have.

Many people will not admit that they are fearful of animals, being alone, being mugged, being stared at, blood, bridges, cancer, choking, crowds, dead bodies, dreams, the dark, death, deformity, dentistry, diseases, drugs, enclosed spaces, failure, fire, fireworks, floods, flying, fog, specific foods, freeways, germs, ghosts, heights, imperfection, inoculations, insects, lightning, medical procedures, meteors, mice, loud noise, open spaces, pain, poison, pregnancy and birth, public speaking, speed, punishment, reptiles, ridicule, roller coasters, sex, sleeping, spiders, strangers, surgery, thunder, vomiting, water, or wounds.

Here's what happened to little Hannah. Liz was making dinner while her five-year-old daughter Hannah was playing in the backyard. She heard a bloodcurdling scream and ran to see what had happened. Hannah was crying hysterically because she had seen a big dog out back. She had developed a fear of dogs after a large one jumped on her when she was only two. Liz said, "I tried everything to comfort her, but I couldn't quiet her, no matter what I did. I was feeling desperate. Then I remembered to use Meridian Therapy on her. After only two rounds she was completely calm."

Overactive Imagination Creates Fear

Sometimes we fear something that hasn't happened but could. Fear of public speaking is the most common fear and stems from anticipation of failure or judgment. Fear of dying, fear of pain, and fear of flying rank high on the list also. Reading about horrendous plane crashes might lead to fantasizing that it could happen to you. When two planes collided over New York City while I was living there, I stopped flying for the next thirty years.

Without ever touching a live snake, you can create a belief that it is slimy and will bite you. Your scared thinking creates a negative reaction that feels real. The same applies to fears of spiders, birds, bats, worms, and other unusual or creepy crawly things.

What Are Phobias?

A phobia is an exaggerated fear, usually inexplicable and illogical. Phobias can create havoc in your life. Avoidance of the thing you fear is always on your mind. In order to avoid what you fear you may even resort to lying to get out of situations that are "dangerous." You might find yourself building your life around your fearfulness. Phobias are often based on real-life frightening experiences of you or someone else you know or have heard about. When that fear gets blown out of proportion, it becomes a phobia. Even though your rational side knows that germs are ever-present, and you have immunity to most diseases, you may still overreact, developing complex rituals and behavior to keep from touching things that might have germs that could contaminate you. Dealing with the dread by using paper towels to touch doorknobs, for instance, then becomes habitual.

Phobias Ruled Their Lives

Jenny hadn't been able to use a public bathroom for more than ten years. As you can imagine, this phobia caused her great inconvenience. After one session of Meridian Therapy with her therapist, she was delighted to be free of this problem. It hasn't returned.

Naomi, a twenty-nine-year-old accountant, had an intense fear of becoming nauseated and vomiting. In college she experienced food poisoning with such severe nausea and vomiting that she felt frightened and powerless. Although most of us have shared a similar event, we have not been permanently affected by it. Naomi's fear became so exaggerated she was extra-wary about what foods were safe to eat and what activities she could participate in that would not upset her equilibrium. Her life was severely restricted as a result of this avoidance pattern. Meridian Therapy freed Naomi from this debilitating condition and gave her freedom to enjoy life.

Fear of Flying

One of the most common fears is fear of flying. Those who fear flying usually focus on distinct aspects of the experience. Fears about the mechanical safety of the plane involve worries about engines failing and disastrous fires. Some people agonize about the pilot's expertise or about pilot error causing a fatal crash. The noise of the engines warming up, the plane's vibrations, and the jolt of leaving the ground or landing may exacerbate the terror. Fears of falling out of the sky, bursting into flames, colliding with another plane, or falling into the ocean all are about dying. These fears may include claustro-phobic fears of being cramped, airsick, or stuck in a closed space for hours while waiting for refueling or waiting in line to take off.

That was Jose's problem. Jose didn't mind being in the air, but he panicked when, after the plane landed, the doors remained closed for what seemed an eternity. He had to fly to Asia and was terrified. He couldn't convince himself that he would get off the plane alive. Jose's realization that the doors would indeed open came after practicing Meridian Therapy for half an hour with me. The fear simply dissolved and he felt as if a huge weight had been lifted.

To address this fear you may want to start with a general approach, referring to the overall problem as "my fear of fly-ing." Rate the degree of discomfort or apprehension you experience *right now* when you think about getting on an air-plane, not how much fear you think you will feel when you fly. Say the affirmation about your fear of flying and proceed to tap. Notice what happens. Perhaps the general sense of anxiety will lessen, or a specific aspect of the fear will emerge. If it does, use the Five Simple Steps you learned in Chapter 2 for that particular aspect. Keep doing this until you have reached a neutral place. Then return to your general fear of flying using the Five Simple Steps. The general approach works, but it may take more time than if you target specific concerns.

The "Stop-Action" Technique

Another way to tackle fear of flying is by breaking the fear down into segments and treating each one. Examine the facets of the experience of traveling by air and notice which ones are upsetting. You can pretend you are watching a movie. Stop the moment you get in touch with a fearful feeling or thought. Tap it until it is gone. Rerun the movie from the beginning. Pause at each anxiety-producing point. Take your time. You don't have to do it all in one sitting. Think about each separate part: preparing for the flight, the airport, before takeoff, on the ground, in the air, and landing.

Take Baby Steps

I often make a list of baby steps with my clients, noting the anxiety rating for each one. Tap them separately until your level of fear reaches zero and you feel no tension in your body. Here is a sample list of anxiety-producing moments.

- Deciding to fly for business or pleasure
- The day before the flight
- The night before the flight
- The day of the flight
- The trip to the airport; arriving at the airport
- Finding the terminal; checking in luggage
- Going through the security check
- Waiting at the gate; hearing the announcement of the flight
- Walking down the walkway or tarmac to the door of the plane
- Stepping into the plane and walking to your seat

- Putting the luggage away
- Fastening the seat belt and looking around
- The flight attendant explaining the safety rules
- Worrying about the competence of the pilot
- The engines starting
- The plane taxis or the plane waits
- Taking off, accelerating, and gaining altitude
- Leveling off and flying at high altitude
- Turbulence
- Descending
- Landing
- Waiting until the doors open

The part of the flight that creates the greatest fear for many flyers is turbulence. Be sure to take time to work on this as well as any other facets of the flying that concern you. Do you mind sitting near the window? Are you anxious when you

Frightened at Coincidences

My neighbor Marion had to make an eleven-hour trip to Europe. She was uncomfortable about flying but became frantic when she realized her flight was scheduled on the anniversary of her mother's death. The pain of her mother's death was still strong in her life. Marion took this as an omen of doom. After a few rounds of tapping she recognized that her rational thinking had replaced her emotional fear. She knew it was just her superstitious beliefs scaring her. A few days later, when asked if she was at all anxious about the coming flight, Marion answered, "I can't be bothered to think about it. It just isn't there."

After spending two wonderful weeks sightseeing, Marion forgot to be anxious about her return trip too. "I wasn't paying attention when the plane took off because I was engrossed in a video game," she said. "When the plane went through turbulence, I experienced a pleasant rocking sensation and wasn't at all afraid." Tapping before the trip had eliminated her fear completely.

are confined in the middle seat? Does the size of the plane cause fear? What about the sounds, smells, and heat or cold you might experience? If you identify with any of these, use Meridian Therapy for each concern.

When the Unexpected Happens

However, there may be times when you will find yourself in a situation you haven't thought to tap about. That is what happened to my colleague Marla when she took a wild ride on a small plane. She related her story:

Just after takeoff the plane started to shake; the turbulence was brutal. I could hear everyone in the plane express their fears by the sounds they were making every time the plane shook. I too was fearful. My thoughts were running wild. Then I had a sudden "aha," and decided to tap. I began by tapping on the fear of flying, but I realized that wasn't really my fear. I like flying. I then tapped on my fear of crashing. In just three rounds things shifted within me. I felt a sudden calmness and began to relax. The plane still shook and rattled. The turbulence was awful, but as I looked out of the window, I just felt as if I was riding a roller coaster, swaying with it, as I enjoyed the rest of the flight. After we landed (on one wheel), I looked around the plane and noticed that people were wiping their brows and sighing with relief. When we complimented the pilot on his good work, he responded, "It doesn't get much worse."

A number of people report using Meridian Therapy to help a seatmate on a plane trip. Joan had overcome her fear of turbulence and was enjoying a trip when the plane began to shudder and jump. The man next to her was obviously upset, so she offered to help him and showed him the points to tap. Lois, another Good Samaritan, aided a young woman before the plane even took off. Her seatmate was scared that she might become airsick. Lois suggested tapping briefly. The girl felt better immediately, and her trip went smoothly.

My Fears About Driving

Most of us do not fly every day, but we often drive daily. Freeway phobias can cause severe stress. I suffered from a twenty-year fear about driving that upset my life. I experienced intense anxiety when my husband drove. My husband is a good driver; it's just that our driving styles are very different. He enjoys speed in the fast lane while I prefer staying in a slower lane. I felt trepidation when, going seventy miles an hour, he would point out things of interest and beautiful scenery instead of looking at the road. I would feel horrified when he zipped over to the exit at the last second or pulled up too close to the car ahead.

As the years progressed my apprehension became more and more severe until it became terror. My unsuccessfully stifled screams alarmed him and interfered with his driving. He didn't appreciate the way I carried on. After a three-hour drive on a vacation trip I had to go to a chiropractor because I had painfully stressed my body by gripping the door handle with my white-knuckled hand. The fear began to make inroads into my life. I avoided visiting friends who lived far away and found excuses not to travel.

During this time I tried a multitude of techniques to over-come the fear: talk therapy, hypnosis, past-life regressions, EMDR, and positive affirmations. Nothing budged the ter-ror. I was in despair. By the time I discovered Meridian Therapy, I was extremely wary and filled with doubt. My introduction to Meridian Therapy was at a training with Dr. Fred Gallo. He helped me remove my fear in half an hour. As the energy points were tapped, dire moments flashed through my mind. I thought about how I dreaded curves in the road, my husband's last-minute rush to the exit, fear of other drivers, and specific scary moments from past trips.

My husband took me for a drive that day to test the results. It was a wonderful experience. As we drove around, I noticed the instances when I would usually make a fear noise or shut my eyes, expecting that to happen again. But it didn't. Actions that previously frightened me were no longer life-or-death moments. It has been years now, and the fear has not returned.

Overcome Your Driving Fears

Some sufferers of highway phobia know which particular aspects of driving cause them to panic. There are drivers who avoid going over bridges or heights; others avoid driving through tunnels or underpasses. Fear of driving in the fast lane, fear of changing lanes, or fear of individual on or off ramps on your particular road system may cause terror.

To overcome driving fears, use the same method I have outlined for fear of flying. You already know exactly what your fear is about. Elise had a problem with narrow roads that curved and wound around and around. Ed was afraid to drive in the rain. If you can't describe what it is that scares you, begin by using the Five Simple Steps for "my fear of driving" or "my fear of the freeway." Perhaps some new thoughts will flit through your mind, suggesting what the components of your fear are. Here are some examples of driving fears.

- I am going to die!
- I will have an accident and be severely injured.
- I don't trust other drivers.
- I'll get lost.
- I can't see in the rain, fog, or dark and will have an accident.
- Someone will rear-end me.
- I'll lose control of my car.
- The driver I'm with will get into an accident.
- I can't handle the curves and will crash.
- Bright lights of oncoming cars will blind me and I'll crash.
- I can't see the lines in the road in the dark or rain.
- I am afraid to pass another car.
- The tunnel will fall in on me.
- The bridge I am on will collapse.
- I will run out of gas and be stranded.

Tap each of your fear thoughts until you reach zero. Then make sure you test yourself by going for a drive.

Eliminate Fear of Heights

Those who suffer from fear of heights will also benefit from Meridian Therapy. Tap your fear away just by thinking about being in a high place, or eliminate the trepidation on the spot. Fear of ladders can be addressed if you or a friend have one on hand. Tap as you look at the ladder. Then climb onto the first step, rate your fear, and tap it away. Continue as you ascend.

As you practice Meridian Therapy to get rid of fear of heights it helps to have a friend assist you. The same holds true for looking over a balcony or out a window many floors above the ground. Although you may overcome your anxiety about looking out the window of a plane, you may still have a terror of elevators, especially the glass ones. Treat each type of height fear separately.

Lions and Tigers and Bears, Oh My!

The story of how Liz helped her terrified daughter overcome her fear of dogs shows how quickly Meridian Therapy can work. Liz told me that a few months after that event, Hannah was on a family outing and didn't flinch when a dog came close by. You can use Meridian Therapy before you are in the vicinity of a dreaded creature, or you can plan to desensitize yourself in its presence. Perhaps you know someone who has a pet dog, cat, rat, hamster, tarantula, or bird you can practice with.

A quick and easy way to end a fear of snakes or lizards is to go to a pet store that carries reptiles and work through your fear right there. It is a good idea to get the cooperation of the store manager during your experiment. Have a friend or support person guide you. If you know your fear originated because someone put a snake on you to scare you when you were in grade school, use Meridian Therapy to defuse that horrible memory first.

When you get to the pet store, begin to treat yourself outside as you anticipate seeing the terrible critters. Use Meridian Therapy for your anxiety about entering the store. Once you are inside and see where they are kept, tap away any fear that arises about going to that part of the store. Proceed slowly, tapping every few feet as you approach the reptile area. Go closer and tap some more. Repeat this process until you are comfortable getting up to the glass cage where the snake or lizard is. Continue to use Meridian Therapy until you are ready to touch and handle it.

Phyllis did this procedure. After forty-five minutes she was handling a lizard without any fear for the first time in her life. In fact, after her trip to the pet store, she decided to go back and get herself a pet lizard.

Get Rid of Your Fear of Dentistry

Dental fears keep many people from getting their teeth attended to. Paul was so wrought up that his dentist had to

It Works for Creepy Crawlies, Too

Thea took away her fear of spiders by tapping. "They gave me the creeps," she said. "If I found one in a cupboard I would be startled. During certain times of the year I would leave the house with a broom in hand making swinging motions in the air as I went down the front stairs to swish their webs away, just in case."

After tapping about her fear she reported, "The next day while walking down the street I watched a black spider crawling kitty-corner across the walkway. I heard myself saying, 'Where are you going, you cute little fellow?' I had to laugh. Never in my life had I had any curiosity about any spider, and cute certainly wasn't ever a word I would have used to describe them!"

give him Valium to quiet him down. Paul learned to tap his fear so the unpleasant quivery feeling in his stomach stopped, and he became calm enough to let the dentist do his work without needing drugs.

One of the most unpleasant dental procedures for many of us is having a dental bite impression made. The feeling of gagging is awful. Some people have a violent gag response. Gagging is a natural protective response, so you won't want to eliminate it entirely. Work with your dentist or hygienist to guide you safely while you tap.

Fear of pain haunted Sandy. When she was a college student she had a traumatic dental experience. She had a root canal performed by a dentist who did not listen when she said that the novocaine wasn't working. He proceeded anyway despite the tears streaming from her eyes. She never forgot the excruciating pain. There was no dental assistant present to help her.

Thirty years later she needed another root canal but was terrified at the thought the same thing would happen again. She used Meridian Therapy to eradicate the early traumatic memory. Next she tapped about her fear of future pain. When she went for the procedure she was calm and unafraid. Sandy was delighted to find that her present practitioner was extremely sympathetic and stopped frequently to check her comfort level.

The Five Simple Steps will address any fear having to do with dentistry. Some patients have trouble sitting in the chair for a routine exam, others fear dental surgery, injections, or extractions. No matter how big or small the issue, you can deal with it. Please let your dentist know what you are doing, so he or she can learn about Meridian Therapy and how it can benefit others.

Go Into Surgery Without Terror

Meridian Therapy can help to quickly relieve fears about surgery. Melina had to have emergency gallbladder surgery. She hadn't much time to prepare, but she quickly treated herself by tapping before going into the operating room. She was able to dispel her fear of dying and found herself joking with the anesthesiologist in a lighthearted way.

Luke, on the other hand, knew when his surgery was to take place. He used tapping beforehand to deal with the anxiety about receiving local anesthetic and went to the hospital feeling so serene he didn't need presurgery medication to calm him. Luke's recovery was so swift he was able to go home much sooner than expected.

This Is Only a Test

Although MRIs are painless, many people react to being enclosed in the tunnel-like compartment. The claustrophobic setting may trigger earlier memories of times you were closed in and felt trapped. Employ the Five Simple Steps to deal with the unpleasant memories before focusing on the MRI.

Medical tests are often pain-free but can be upsetting in other ways. When Jamie heard about a new diagnostic-imaging test for breast tumors that might help her, she was excited. She had a large benign tumor that worried her doctors. The imaging machinery did not enclose her like the MRI. However, she had to lie in a very uncomfortable position, teetering on top of a pile of narrow pillows for twenty minutes, without moving. "I was twisted like a pretzel," she said. "I could feel my arms begin to quiver from the strain of holding still. I was terrified that if I moved they might make me do it all over again, and I knew I couldn't keep that pose again. I imagined tapping the points over and over and made it through."

Most people understand how common the fear of needles is. Receiving injections or having blood drawn is terrifying to many children and adults. Melina said, "Before Meridian Therapy when I had to have needles or blood drawn the fear was so intense I felt like I was dying. Now I am not afraid."

Help Frightened Infants

I can remember how harrowing it was to go to the pediatrician for a checkup or shots when my children were babies.

You can't explain to a six-month-old that it will only hurt for a second. How splendid it is that a parent can tap herself as a surrogate or tap her child to reassure, quiet the fear, and avoid having a screaming baby to contend with.

Meridian Therapy helped an eight-day-old baby go through a painful ritual. Larry was asked to hold his newborn nephew during the baby's bris (ritual circumcision) and give the baby a traditional wine-dipped cloth to suck during the ceremony. Larry described what occurred.

"I decided to tap my nephew throughout the procedure. Even before giving the wine, whenever he started to get uncomfortable, I tapped on the Eyebrow point, sang to him, and told him that I loved him. I tapped pretty much through the entire ceremony. He hardly cried at all. It was quite apparent to everyone there that this boy was unusually calm."

Afraid of Santa

Meridian Therapy can help children with many kinds of fears. Here is a firsthand report from a caring parent who was able to help someone else's child.

I have just returned from a Christmas party for the kids in a weekly playgroup. Last year the kids were all about two to three years old and meeting Santa was, for many of them, a bit of a challenge. Most were overwhelmed, many cried, and some wouldn't go near this strange man in the red suit, even after frantic attempts by parents to pacify them. This year, with the kids a year older, we fully expected it to be different. Most of the kids were excitedly looking forward to seeing Santa, having learned the association between Santa and presents, except for Karen.

As we stood waiting for Santa to arrive, Karen's mother told me she was frightened to the point of near hysteria by the thought of Santa. I hastily explained the tapping formula treatment. I suggested she tap her daughter a few times before Santa arrived and again when he was there.

As Santa made his way down the path a few minutes later, I saw the very upset, frightened little girl run into her mother's arms. I saw the mother with a worried look, trying desperately to do the tapping, then holding her girl tight. A minute later, leaving Karen with her father, the mother came to tell me it "didn't work," and her daughter was still very upset.

I pointed toward the front of the group, where her husband was now walking with Karen toward Santa, holding hands. We watched as Karen walked up to Santa with a smile on her face, accepted a gift from him, and even paused for a while to talk to him, smiling happily as she did so. You should have seen the proud, relieved faces on both her parents. I paused for a while to give thanks to God, and to those who have passed on the gift of this tapping technique that allowed this miracle to happen. What greater gift can we give than this, to relieve a little girl's pain and turn it to joy.

Teach the Little Ones to Tap

Parents, teachers, grandparents, babysitters, and friends can help children who are afraid or hurting. Sharon, a therapist who practices Meridian Therapy, helped her six-year-old granddaughter Cheri overcome swimming fears. Grandma had the girl say, "Even though I think I'll never be able to swim as well as I'd like, I love myself just the way I am and I'm OK." After the swimming lesson, the teacher told Sharon that Cheri was the only one who hadn't been afraid to jump into the pool.

Use Meridian Therapy when a child has a scary nightmare, right then, to allay the fear. Jack says his four-year-old son drifts off to sleep after only one round of tapping. When children are small, you can cuddle them and tap yourself as a surrogate while you talk about their upset. Make Meridian Therapy a game or sing about the fear as you tap the child. Children can learn to tap themselves too. Your child will feel better and so will you.

The majority of people find that once they eliminate a fear or phobia with Meridian Therapy it does not return. Now that you know how easy it is to erase your fears by tapping them away, you can get started immediately.

chapter seven

Turn "Never" into "Now": Overcome Procrastination

Procrastinators put off doing things, wait till the last minute, and then hate themselves for not completing projects or assignments. Do you find yourself making excuses for procrastinating? Dieters always say they will start on Monday. How many times have you said, "I'll do it, but first I want to watch this basketball game, finish this chapter, make a phone call, or go to the store before it closes"? "I'm too tired" and "There's not enough time" are other reasons for postponing. When asked why he was dragging his feet about finishing a term paper, Darryl, a twenty-year-old college student, explained, "I'm young; there's time." Excuses cloud the real reason you want to wait, which is *fear*.

Procrastination is not just a bad habit, it is an unsuccessful way of coping with anxiety or fear. Everyone procrastinates at some time or knows someone who does. Many procrastinators are perfectionists. I have been treating procrastinators and perfectionists from all walks of life for twenty years. Meridian Therapy addresses the underlying issues that keep you stuck in procrastination and perfectionism.

The way you act, what you do or don't do, is a direct response to your emotions. If you feel happy, your actions reflect that. When you feel sad, mad, or scared, your behavior mirrors those moods, too. Fear is the usual source of putting off or waiting. Telling yourself to "tough it out" or "just do it" doesn't work because the unconscious fear is so paralyzing that you are willing to take the consequences of putting things off, rather than know what the real dread is and face it. Anthony had to repeat a semester of college because he wouldn't hand in papers that weren't "perfect." Numerous Americans delay completing their tax returns, even though the result is a hefty penalty. Putting off a trip to the dentist because you are afraid you will need expensive or painful procedures may result in needing them because you waited too long.

Five Fears That Stop Procrastinators

Here is a list of five important fears procrastinators react to:

1. Fear of failure
2. Fear of judgment
3. Fear of success
4. Fear of authority
5. Fear of the future

These fears pervade the lives of people who operate from an unconscious worry about what others will think. Meridian Therapy helps transform the negative feelings that trigger procrastination and perfectionism into positive action.

Childhood Beginnings

The roots of procrastination begin to grow in childhood. Most children are under pressure both at home and at school. Adults give messages about how to act, indicating, "People won't like you if you _____." These statements seem like commandments from God to a child and translate into the *shoulds* and *should nots* that still plague most of us. Teachers demand that assignments be in on time. Parents want kids to clean their room, put away clothing and toys, and do whatever they say to be acceptable or "good."

A child with shaky self-confidence begins to delay completing tasks because he is afraid he won't be good enough. At school, he doesn't finish a report because he imagines the grade will be unsatisfactory, and he doesn't want to find out he is as stupid as he supposes. This pattern becomes habitual if not broken.

When I teach classes about overcoming procrastination, I tell my students there is no such thing as lazy. Lazy is what *they* label you when you don't do what they want you to do. Most of us are rarely lazy when it comes to something we love or truly want.

Guilt Trips Galore

Read these common parental mandates. Each one is certain to make you feel guilty, if you believe it. Which ones do you still cling to? For every statement you are still restricted by, practice the Five Simple Steps until you no longer agree.

- People won't like you if you speak out of turn.
- People won't like you if you aren't good enough.

- People won't like you if you call attention to yourself.
- People won't like you if you are too good, talented, or good-looking.
- People won't like you if you disagree with them.
- People won't like you if you get dirty.
- People won't like you if you break the rules.
- People won't like you if you aren't perfect.

Can you think of some I haven't listed? Write them down. Focus on one at a time, tapping each one until you are free of any negative emotional charge.

Each of the five fears operates on a subconscious level, and misery and failure are often the result. Here are some examples from the lives of procrastinators I have helped.

1. Fear of Failure

Fear of failure pervades our lives. Some people won't ask for directions when they are lost because they are afraid they will seem foolish. How many of us have unfinished projects in the closet or garage, left there because they might not be good enough when completed?

Melissa, a new Tupperware representative, was about to lead her first gathering and kept putting off preparing her presentation. The day before the event she was so frustrated at her procrastination she began to tap about not being ready. Here is what unfolded:

Round One: I remember a time years ago when my sister Sheri forced me to do a talk in front of a group of her friends. I was so scared I became tongue-tied and embarrassed.

Round Two: I can hear my family saying, "You can't do anything right. You make a fool of yourself."

Round Three: I feel a pain in my chest.

Round Four: I hear a voice saying, "Why did you cause me pain?"

Round Five: I see myself as a child, on my knees crying. I feel humiliated.

Round Six: I am in a corner. I don't want anyone to see me.

Round Seven: I am afraid.

Round Eight: I remember my sister being angry with me because I was nervous.

Round Nine: She says I'm a dingbat. I'm stupid and worthless.

Round Ten: If Sheri is angry, it's her problem.

Round Eleven: I don't believe I'm stupid and worthless!

Round Twelve: I feel OK now.

While Melissa was tapping about not being ready for tomorrow, old memories came to light. Some were vague, but a specific recollection about Sheri reminded her of feelings of inadequacy. After dealing with this problem, Melissa went on to do a fine job the next day and received many compliments about her presentation.

2. Fear of Judgment by Others

Fear of judgment by others motivates most of us and is at the heart of perfectionism. Perfectionists are not born that way; society creates them. When you are obsessed about what other people think, you create a life of bondage to outside validation.

Goro Yamaguchi was a famous Japanese musician who cared little for fame. He said, comparing himself to a flower, "People may look at me, or they may not. I will still bloom." How many of us can say that?

The Pain of Perfectionism

The main negative belief perfectionists dwell on is, "It won't be good enough." They translate it as, "I'm not good enough." Perfectionists suffer from constant stress because of their irrational ideas. Critical thoughts and beliefs create and feed the fear of judgment. These convictions are guaranteed to create anxiety if you think they are true.

- People will think I am stupid if I make a mistake.
- People will laugh at me.
- Average isn't good enough.
- I have to do it *right* (perfectly).
- If I can't do something well, there is little point in doing it.

- I should be upset if I make a mistake.
- If I work hard enough, I should be able to excel at anything I try.
- Failing at something important means I am less of a person.

Which of the negative perfectionistic beliefs do you identify with? Use tapping to transform each one. Remember the times you were hampered or paralyzed by a situation or relationship because of your fear of looking foolish or being "average." Tap to release each memory and forgive yourself. Acknowledge and accept everything that comes to mind. Perhaps you will feel sad or mad. If you start to feel a bodily sensation for which you have no words, tap on that heaviness in your heart or the lump in your throat. Tap until you feel neutral.

What Others Think Is None of Your Business!

If, like Ben, you are worried about what others will think, tap as you describe the situation. Say, "Even though I care what my father thinks, and I fear his disapproval, I deeply and completely accept myself." Tap as you remind yourself, "Father's opinion matters to me;" or "I am afraid of his criticism." Do this for each person you have given power to upset you.

Finally, test yourself by stating the negative belief in a loud voice: "I am afraid they will laugh at me!" Is there any upset left? Did an additional thought or unhappy memory arise? Continue until you feel free of the burden of your belief. Fear of what others think will inevitably surface at different times in your life. Each time you become aware that you are acquiescing to others' opinions, tap until you decide what to do about it.

Writer's Block Stopped Him

Ben, a successful writer, stopped in the middle of writing a book, unable to motivate himself. While tapping to overcome his writer's block, one of the first things he realized was that his problem began right after a disagreement with his editor. The editor's criticism of Ben's work started him wondering if he were really good enough. As he tapped he understood that he was afraid he would be laughed at when his book was published. People might think he had no talent. The public wouldn't buy his book, and his writing career would be over.

Ben kept thinking of all the people who had high expectations of him. I asked him to name the individuals whose criticism he feared. I was surprised when he didn't name any literary critics. He was most worried about the reactions of his parents and friends. Then I asked him what qualified them to judge him. He was taken aback by my question. Ben realized he was the one who had given them the power to judge him. Tapping about his fear opened up many memories of previous embarrassing events and concerns about his vulnerability. He tapped, focusing on each person he feared, until he no longer cared what they thought. Once the burden of fear was gone, he began to write again.

3. Fear of Success

Winning the lottery is something many people like to imagine. I counsel people who, even though they say they want love, fame, fortune, and happiness, are afraid of having it all. They undermine themselves by procrastinating. Putting off getting skills training, putting off going for interviews, and finding excuses not to put their best foot forward keep them stuck and unhappy.

Surf's Up

Stephen, a college athlete, was a talented surfer. Even though he was outstanding, there were two other men on his team who usually beat him. Stephen trained hard and loved sports, yet he didn't perform the way he knew he could. First, Stephen thought he was holding himself back because he had some anxiety about big waves. He tapped about the waves and soon brought his discomfort to zero. Next, he remembered he felt funny at the top of a big wave, looking down, and that, too, was easily dealt with.

To test himself, Stephen thought about the coming meet the next weekend. He imagined the big waves and surfing on top of a tall one. He felt good, but a voice within said, "I'm not supposed to win." He was shocked, because he had always thought of himself as a competitor. After tapping for a few minutes he felt completely confident. That weekend he won over his two opponents.

You Deserve It!

If you suffer from fear of success, ask yourself if you deserve to succeed. If you think you have a fear of success, you may have a problem about worthiness. What do you secretly believe you don't deserve? One way to find out how you are stopping yourself is to engage in the following activity.

1. On the top of a paper write "I deserve _____."
   Finish the sentence with whatever seems to be
   out of your reach. For example:

   > I deserve love.

   > I deserve money.

   > I deserve a new job.

   > I deserve friends.

   > I deserve happiness.

   > I deserve health.

2. Say your affirmation out loud. Then say,
   "No I don't because . . ." or, "Yes, but . . ."
   Write down the first negative thought that
   springs to mind.
3. Tap while stating the self-effacing thought
   out loud until it dissipates or you replace it
   with a positive alternative.
4. Repeat the original affirmation, listening for
   a new rebuttal each time. Tap the negative
   "Yes buts" until you run out of them. Finally
   say your affirmation aloud with feeling.

After you have completed this exercise, ask yourself what
you are going to do immediately to move toward success. List
three things you are willing to spend at least fifteen minutes
doing this week to achieve your goal. If you can't think of
three things or if you don't follow through with the ones you
chose, use Meridian Therapy to tap away your excuses. Look
for additional thoughts or beliefs holding you back. Don't
give up. Persistence will win out.

4. Fear of Authority

One of the most common reasons for procrastination is rebellion against those in charge. We are all familiar with the two-year-old who says no to everything. Power struggles are part of child development. One of the ways children rebel against authority is by dragging their feet or "forgetting." It can be a way to say no without words. When you are small, those in command are your parents, teachers, ministers, and other grownups. Who is the authority you are rebelling against when you put off cleaning the garage or paying your bills? If you are an adult with your own home, job, spouse, and family, who must you obey?

You may be the unhappy servant of the parent within. That inner critic is the guilt producer, the one whose commandments are *should* and *shouldn't*. When you use *should, must, have to* and *ought to*, you really mean, *I don't want to but they're making me!* These words create guilt in many adults who drag their feet as a way of rebelling. The more you delay, the more you are shamed by the *shoulds*. The result is a load of guilt.

No matter how old you are, *shoulds* keep you a child. The inner child doesn't want to do her chores now. The child wants to watch TV or relax. Putting things off is another way of thumbing your nose at "them." Adults don't need *shoulds*. *Shoulds* are for children. Using *shoulds* is the way we teach our young how to be part of our society. If that is true, how will you get rid of your *shoulds?* By tapping, of course.

What Melissa Discovered

Melissa, the Tupperware representative I described earlier, worried about her problem with time commitments. She frequently arrived late and canceled appointments for no reason other than a feeling that she just didn't want to go. She said, "I hate to make a promise about meeting people. I balk at the thought of having to show up at a designated time. I experience dread when I *have to* do something." As she tapped about her frustration, Melissa felt a great deal of anger. First she tapped about authority in general. Soon she released anger toward the demands of her father, her mother, and her former boss. Rebellion had cost her too much. She now knew that no one was making her do anything. The choice was hers alone.

Taming Your Temper Tantrum

What are you putting off that you *should* be doing and deep down don't want to? Make a list. Include the obvious chores like cooking, cleaning, fixing, paying bills, writing letters, and returning phone calls or e-mails. Ask yourself what else you don't want to do that you are putting off. Maybe you are procrastinating because you want to say "No" to people and are afraid of hurting their feelings. Were you taught to squelch your own beliefs or emotions so as not to hurt others?

Employ Meridian Therapy for each thing you are currently not doing and feel guilty about. You can tap "garage guilt" if you still haven't tackled that cleaning job. "I should write that letter." "I have to go to my cousin's wedding and I don't want to." "I should pay my bills on time." "Guilty about breaking my dental appointment." Make up your own version.

When Tania used Meridian Therapy because she was far behind in completing a report at work, she discovered that her inner-child self was tired of working. Although Tania liked her work, her inner child just wanted to play and be irresponsible. Tapping helped Tania reconsider her schedule to balance work and play. She began to make more time for having fun and relaxing as well as attending to business.

As adults we frequently do things we don't particularly want to, like drive a car pool, pay taxes, work overtime, and stop at red lights when no cars are in sight. After tapping you may notice you have decided to do the chore or activity, but without guilt. Conversely, you may decide that you aren't going to do the laundry, clean your car, or spend time with someone you don't like. Perhaps as you tap you will come up with creative solutions that surprise you.

Discipline Is a Dirty Word

Jeff, a forty-five-year-old who was working and taking classes at night, drove himself to be perfect. He worked hard to complete a task, only to find that there were too many more things to be done and not enough time. He constantly felt guilty and unworthy. Jeff thought that he needed to discipline himself more. At the same time, the word discipline brought up rage and a feeling of being punished. Jeff liked to exercise but didn't follow through because he would need to be disciplined to achieve his goal and the "D" word was like a red flag.

He treated the quandary of this double bind with Meridian

Therapy. What emerged was a cycle of feelings that alternated between anger and hurt. He tapped until he felt a glimmer of hope that there was light at the end of the tunnel. Jeff announced, "No one is making me do anything. I have a choice." After that, Jeff began to exercise more. He kept at it even when some of the anger arose. "I just tap it away," he said.

When you eliminate the *should*s and *have to*s, you will be able to replace them with *choose to* or *choose not to*. That is what Jeff did. The most important result of this exercise is that guilt will disappear. If you don't believe me, try it and see.

5. Fear of the Future

If you have read this far and still aren't clear about what your fears are, perhaps you are putting off doing something now in order to avoid what you will face in the near future, after you complete the task.

Ed, single again after an unhappy marriage, was renovating his house. He kept putting off finishing the cabinets in his kitchen. Although he had redone his entire house except for this last project, he kept dragging his feet and couldn't figure out why. When he practiced Meridian Therapy he realized that if his house were complete, he would have to invite people over, begin to socialize, and maybe get married again. There is no relationship between home remodeling and getting married, except in Ed's convoluted thinking. As he tapped he realized that he could finish the cabinets and also stay single, if he chose.

We all participate in this kind of twisted thinking at some time. You can challenge your irrational convictions by interrogating yourself as you tap the energy points. Ask this question: "What am I *afraid* will happen if I complete this project?" After you get an answer, ask yourself, "Then what am I afraid will happen?" Keep asking and answering until you get to the root of the problem. That's what Elaine did.

The "What Am I Afraid Of" Dialogue

Elaine, a forty-year-old single woman, complained that she couldn't make herself clean her house. She hated the mess but busied herself with other activities that kept her on the run rather than straighten up her small apartment. Here is what she discovered as she used the "What am I afraid of" dialogue while tapping.

Q: What am I afraid will happen if I clean my home?
A: I will have to do it all by myself.

Q: What am I afraid will happen if I do it all by myself?
A: I will feel angry and resentful.

Q: What am I afraid will happen if I feel angry and resentful?
A: I will realize that no one is taking care of me.

Q: What am I afraid will happen if no one takes care of me?
A: I will have to face my mother's death. She took care of me, and then she died and left me. She will never take care of me again. I will be alone forever.

Elaine's thinking was irrational. She believed that if she cleaned her house, it meant accepting that her beloved mother was never coming back to take care of her. Putting off cleaning was a way of putting off acknowledging the finality of her loss. She tapped about her inability to deal with the loss. When she reached zero, she let go of her twisted thinking. After that, she happily cleaned her apartment.

Become a Former Procrastinator

The dynamics underlying procrastination are complex. There may be other fears hindering you from completing projects. Meridian Therapy will help you uncover many aspects of this self-defeating behavior. Keep reminding yourself to look for the fear that you are hiding from yourself. Through regular tapping, you can turn your fearful beliefs into positive attitudes that lead to successful action.

chapter eight

Conquer Cravings and Compulsions

If you can't control when you start or when you stop a behavior or using a substance, you have a problem called compulsion. Compulsion is a sign of a life out of balance. Fulfilling unstoppable cravings often becomes addictive. Addicts continue to abuse substances and overdo behavior despite the negative consequences. When they try to stop they experience the pain of withdrawal. People addicted to alcohol, drugs, and caffeine become ill when they try to stop. Compulsive exercisers, overeaters, and those whose habits don't involve chemical substances suffer from a different kind of withdrawal. They feel intense anxiety or irritability when they are deprived of their "medication."

Over the years I have collected a long list of activities and substances other than alcohol and drugs that people can't say no to. My clients include people who are unable to control their behavior toward food, cigarettes, caffeine, shopping, sex, gambling, exercising, working, watching soap operas, computer games, Internet sex, computer chat rooms, reading, collecting, sewing, gardening, golfing, watching sports, shoplifting, gum chewing, licking lip balms, hair cutting, self cutting, committing crimes, masturbating, doing crafts, hobbies, and packratting. One woman was even addicted to worrying. What do all these people have in common? They are unable to cope with intense stress, so they turn to these activities in an attempt to soothe themselves.

Stress and Your Brain

I believe in the equation *stress equals craving*. So does Dr. Ronald Ruden, author of *The Craving Brain*, who has spent years working with food and drug addicts. He maintains that the roots of craving lie in the brain. When dopamine and serotonin, two important neurotransmitters, become unbalanced, there is a complex chain reaction in ancient survival mechanisms in the brain. When dopamine rises, the brain sends a message, "I gotta have it." Dopamine helps us focus and drives us toward a goal, while serotonin creates the feeling of completion and satisfaction when we get what we are after.

Ruden points out that three factors can cause this imbalance: genes, hormones, and stress. When dopamine is high, serotonin is too low to create the "Yes, I got it!" sensation. The person keeps experiencing the "I gotta have it" urge without ceasing. That is why addicts say, "One is never enough and a dozen is not too many." The addict keeps feeling the "I gotta have it" despite discomfort and misery that can even lead to death. Reaction to stress affects the activity of dopamine and serotonin in the brain.

The Craving Cycle

In my books about eating and spending disorders, *A Substance Called Food* and *Born to Spend*, I tell readers that a binge is a temper tantrum characterized by the thought "Ain't it awful, and there's nothing I can do about it!" You feel impotent when an unpleasant situation or relationship is prolonged or irritating. The feeling of frustration leads to greater anger that culminates with a binge. I call this Super Stress.

During Super Stress the craving cycle is activated. The memory of the reward makes the addict seek that joyful state over and over again. Compulsive people react not only to alcohol, food, or drugs, but to other cues, such as reading an ad for alcohol, smelling food outside a restaurant, seeing a syringe, or thinking about a holiday associated with food or drink. These triggers set off the compulsive pursuit of gratification that turns into insatiable craving and the inability to stop.

It is clear that compulsive activities relieve anxiety in the craving brain. Pleasurable activities like spending, eating, gambling, and escaping from worries by spending hours at the computer also mask the pain of the problems of living. The substance or behavior soon seems to be a solution to all problems. Life problems become harder to cope with as stress accumulates year after year. Meridian Therapy tapping will reduce your stress level and allow you to solve problems that appear to be unyielding. You can use Meridian Therapy to eliminate all sorts of cravings and help prevent binges.

A Weekend with Grandma

Marilyn wanted to give up smoking, but didn't know how to cope when she spent weekends with her difficult, aged grandmother, a heavy smoker. Grandmother loved her daily predinner ritual of cocktails and cigarettes, and Marilyn admitted she did too. It was hard to go against her grandmother's demands. The relationship was tense because the old woman was very needy and difficult to get along with.

Marilyn tapped about her upcoming visit, focusing on her smoking problem. She also tapped about how she was giving up satisfying her own needs to please her grandmother. Soon she was able to imagine herself acting strong during her visit. Despite the tapping Marilyn gave in to the enticement of alcohol and cigarettes on the first night of her visit. Undaunted, she continued to tap about her frustrations. The following night she was able to resist temptation. Not only that, she also ate less junk food during her stay.

Relieving Smokers' Depression

Of all the substances people become addicted to, cigarettes are unique because the nicotine has an antidepressant quality. When those who smoke more than two packs a day try to stop, they frequently become depressed and go back to smoking. Marilyn also had to deal with her depressed mood as she eliminated cigarettes. Tapping helped her rethink beliefs that kept her stuck in negativity and hopelessness.

Meridian Therapy will not eliminate addiction or compulsion outright. It can take away cravings for specific substances and activities and will provide you with the means to resolve particular problems that create the Super Stress that leads to unstoppable cravings. Test the results for yourself with the Craving Challenge.

The Craving Challenge

Try this experiment with chocolate. Almost everyone has a taste for chocolate. You most likely will have something chocolate in your home right now, a piece of candy, a cookie, or cake. If sweets are not what you crave, you may want to challenge your desire for a cigarette or beer instead.

- Hold the chocolate item in your hand. Smell it.
- Take a very small bite and savor it.
- Rate the intensity of your desire to eat it right now on a scale of zero to ten.
- Use the Meridian Therapy affirmation and tapping sequence.
- Hold the chocolate in your hand. Smell it again.
- Rate the intensity of your craving. Has it changed?
- Use the Meridian Therapy sequence again.
- Continue to tap and rate your desire until you have reached zero.
- You will want to discard the rest of the uneaten food.

You will be amazed at how quickly the craving for chocolate dissipates, often after only one or two rounds. Many people report that the aroma changes, becoming less appealing. Use the craving challenge with cigarettes, alcohol, or coffee. Use it with urges to spend and any other impulses you are troubled about. Alcoholics and drug abusers must abstain completely from these drugs. However, Meridian Therapy makes abstinence easier. One day at a time can add up to years.

If, instead of feeling less and less like eating the chocolate, your craving increased, you may have gotten in touch with an upsetting thought or memory that is somehow related to your desire. Begin with the new idea or emotion and use the Five Simple Steps until you reach zero. Then return to the chocolate and rate the strength of your craving. Keep tapping about the craving and any other aspects that arise until the urge is gone.

It Isn't Painful

Let's assume you like green beans and eat them occasionally. When you don't have green beans in the house, do you become anxious and irritated? Do you have to go to the market to make sure you get a fresh supply? Or do you eat spinach instead and feel just as satisfied? You don't feel deprived because you know you can have green beans again, if you want them. Maybe you don't want them today. Using Meridian Therapy you can achieve this feeling of freedom from the tyranny of craving.

My Chocolate Miracle

Most people who have used Meridian Therapy to combat cravings report a loss of desire that lasts for hours, days, or longer. Sometimes the craving is extinguished permanently. This is what happened to me. More than three years ago I received a gift of a glorious box of very expensive chocolates. It was very tempting. I didn't want to open this Pandora's box, so I put it on a table where it proceeded to beckon me. I couldn't live with it, but I couldn't live without it either.

Since I specialize in helping people overcome their compulsions, I did what I tell my clients to do. I gave myself a two-minute treatment using Meridian Therapy, tapping the energy points while agonizing over my desire for those luscious pieces of chocolate. My urge to gobble them up quickly dissipated. I expected that after tapping successfully to control my craving I would be free of wanting chocolate *for that day*. However, I had no intention of living my life without chocolate. During the next four days I continued to tap my energy points two or three times a day, all the while looking lovingly at the golden box. I didn't open it.

By the fifth day it began to dawn on me that I had lost interest in the candy. As the days turned into weeks, I noticed that I had not only stopped craving the gift box of chocolate, I stopped desiring chocolate entirely. It happened so easily that I was sure it wouldn't last. It has been more than three years and the old unstoppable craving hasn't returned yet! Now I am truly, effortlessly free, thanks to Meridian Therapy. Freedom means sometimes I eat chocolate and sometimes I don't, and it's no big deal. It's no different from eating or not eating green beans.

1-2-3 Safety or Danger Scale

Super Stress creates craving, and compulsion is all about giving in to cravings. Compulsive people are often not aware of the connection. All they feel is an urge for *that something*. Mostly when people say they are under stress, they mean they are either scared or mad. Here is an easy way to judge how stressful particular situations in your life may be. I call it the 1-2-3 Safety or Danger Scale.

One stands for any experience or relationship that is stress-free. When you think about it, you feel no concern, no butterflies in your stomach or tightening in your body. A rating of *three* is for something so overwhelming that you can't cope with it at this time. A *three* will almost certainly cause you to go out of control. A rating of *two* means maybe I can handle it and maybe I can't.

When you are confronted with a situation, take a moment to ask yourself if it is physically and emotionally safe or dangerous for you. You won't have any trouble with the *ones*. Use Meridian Therapy to turn *twos* into *ones*. Tap to follow through with a *three* and transform it into a *two* or a *one*.

Evaluating your options in this simple way will teach you to be more aware of yourself. If you overestimate your state of mind and find that a *two* is really a *three*, instead of berating yourself, do a postmortem on your unsuccessful experience. What was hard for you? At what point did your anxiety get out of hand? Learn from what didn't work, and you will be able to avoid putting yourself in harm's way in the future. That is what Nicole did.

When Things Don't Go Your Way

After her divorce Nicole, a problem drinker, was lonely. She was invited to a party given by a friend and discovered that her ex-husband would also be there with his new girlfriend. Nicole truly believed she would be okay. Seeing people, including her ex, with partners and having fun, while she was dateless, turned out to be overwhelming. She became so upset, she thought she would burst into tears in front of everyone. Nicole went into the bathroom and used Meridian Therapy to calm her intense feelings. As she tapped, she realized that if she stayed and tried to be "strong," she would drink. She made her excuses and left early. Instead of getting high, she felt good about taking care of herself. When she went home, she phoned her AA sponsor for support.

Super Stress results when things don't go the way you want them to. Somehow the world isn't following your script. The more you struggle to get what you want, the more powerless you feel when it doesn't work. Anyone who is in a twelve-step program is familiar with the idea that you must admit you are powerless over your substance or behavior in order to succeed. A binge reflects the amount of frustration about all the things in your life you feel unable to change.

When you are thinking, "Ain't it awful, and there's nothing I can do about it," the "it" isn't alcohol, drugs, food, cigarettes, sex, or spending. The "it" that is driving you up the wall can be your boss, your kids, a cranky spouse, a car that needs new tires, the weather, Christmas, paying bills, a broken heart, the plumber who is late, a computer crash, forgetting a promise, and many other big and small things in your life.

Sam's Story

Sam, a single man turning fifty, was a very unhappy beer drinker who was in denial about his alcoholism. He would often come home and drink a six-pack of beer in the evening. Before long, he realized his drinking was becoming a problem. One wintry day I saw Sam after work and asked him if he intended to drink beer that evening. He answered "Yes." I asked if he would be interested in trying Meridian Therapy as an experiment. I explained that even though Meridian Therapy might take away his craving, the choice was his whether he went home and drank or not.

Sam wasn't sure he wanted to forgo his beer, but agreed to go along with Meridian Therapy. As he tapped, he became less and less interested in the beer. Finally, Sam said, "I wouldn't mind a bowl of hot soup. Yes, that would hit the spot." Sam was certainly surprised at the switch. It seemed to happen without his trying to make it happen. In fact, he hadn't really wanted to stop craving beer at all.

Why the Beer Won

Although when he was in my office Sam really wanted soup more than beer, once he was home he reverted to his nightly binge. Sam's Super Stress hadn't been addressed. One of his major miseries was about where he lived. He suffered from the noise of the nearby highway and the dismal view. If that weren't enough, Sam hated his job but didn't feel qualified for much else. "I'm too old to change," he kept saying. There didn't seem much to live for. He felt powerless over everything!

Cravings are an indication of intense negative emotion. Sam had a choice, but he didn't know it. He could either pay attention to the situation creating stress, or ignore it and soothe himself with alcohol. After the spree the problem was still there the next morning. With continued tapping, Sam began to address his underlying issues. As he made new decisions about valuing himself, getting into a new line of work, and moving to a more desirable location, he realized that he could let go of excessive drinking and made plans to join a support group.

Getting Your Power Back

Employ the Daily Workout described in Chapter 3. Tap about everyone and everything you feel powerless over. Do this at least once a day. Tap about the substance or behavior you crave as often as possible. If you tap for one minute ten times a day you will certainly see results.

Compulsive people tend to discount their feelings. Maybe you aren't letting yourself know how much you are bothered, angered, saddened, disappointed, or frightened. Have you ever told yourself, "I can handle that," but later felt out of sorts and developed a headache, picked a fight with your spouse, or had a binge? Finally you admitted to yourself you didn't "handle" the situation very well. You overestimated your ability or emotional strength, just as Nicole did in going to the party where she would see her ex-husband. Daily tapping will enable you to honor the power within that can help you solve your problems.

Tap Away Your Cravings

Many people who crave alcohol, drugs, cigarettes, food, sex, or spending believe that the only way to resist is through the white-knuckle willpower method, cold turkey, or a twelve-step program. If you are in a recovery program or psychotherapy, Meridian Therapy will enhance your progress. Practicing tapping can make cravings disappear effortlessly. You can begin to test its effectiveness when you have a specific craving by using the Five Simple Steps when you are in the presence of temptation or contemplating something you'll regret later.

Cravings can also be avoided if you tap when you are not in the throes of desire. All you have to do is think about how you crave something and tap the energy points as you speak of your problem—"sugar craving," "can't resist eBay auctions," or "the second glass of wine." It is easier to tap when your dopamine isn't up and the "I gotta have it" feeling hasn't taken over. Think about your cravings and tap for one minute as often as you can throughout the day. You will be delighted with the results.

Charles decided to try a system of tapping four times a day to control his craving for wine. There was no effect for the first two weeks, but he didn't give up. At week five he felt totally in control of how much he drank. He noticed that he would only drink two glasses of wine or beer during the evening because after two it didn't taste the same anymore, and he lost interest.

Juice Abuse

Jo was puzzled about eating large amounts when she wasn't really hungry or thirsty, so she came to see me because she was desperate to control her urges and lose weight. Jo extinguished her cravings despite herself. One of Jo's favorite foods was juice. Because she came from a very large family that couldn't afford juice except as a treat, Jo adored it. She could drink a quart at one sitting.

As we talked, I asked her if she might consider having juice but drinking less every day. I could see from her face that she was struggling to maintain her adult rational state while the child self within obviously wanted to rebel. I asked Jo to tell me what she really thought of my suggestion. She answered, "No way!" in a loud, angry voice.

I asked her to use Meridian Therapy and say "No way" in that rebellious, furious voice. Instead of her anger lessening, Jo got more enraged as she tapped. She wasn't thinking about juice. Other aspects of her eating compulsion came to light. Jo saw that her intense craving wasn't for food but for someone to pay attention to her. Her mother had died when she was a baby. She was the youngest and was forgotten and neglected by her stepmother. She grieved as she said, "If my mom were alive, she would have taken care of me. It's not fair."

Jo was relieved to see the connection between her sad and abused childhood and a hunger that could never be satisfied. She still wasn't sure about the juice. Then a wonderful thing happened. Jo ran out of juice one day and forgot to buy more. She had no desire for it. Jo continued to use tapping for many of the stresses in her life. By the end of a year she had lost more than twenty pounds. Two years have elapsed and she is still not interested in drinking large quantities of juice.

On-the-Spot Tapping

Practice Meridian Therapy on the spot. An exciting way to face temptation head-on is go to a restaurant, shopping mall, or bar where you can feel the craving. You will need the help of someone you can trust who is free from compulsive problems. Tell your companion you are going to perform an experiment. This person needs to be supportive and not make judgmental comments. It is even more helpful if your friend taps along with you. Set a limit for how much time you will spend there. Once you have arrived, follow these instructions.

- Tap before you enter the place you have chosen. Rate your craving or anxiety, then tap to take the edge off your stress.
- After you are inside, look around. Are you anxious, fearful, excited, tempted? Share some of your thoughts or feelings with your helper. Using Narrative Meridian Therapy, tap as you talk.
- If you are in a restaurant, read the menu and tap any cravings. In a bar, think about what you would like to drink and tap about the desire. If you are in a mall, pick a store and tap about your urges to shop as you walk around different departments trying on clothes or touching merchandise. Become aware of triggers, sounds, smells, or people you associate with the rush to satisfy your craving.
- Leave the place when your time is up, and go to a quiet spot. Take stock of your adventure. What happened? What did you learn? What will you do now? Ask your companion for feedback.

Remember the equation *stress equals craving*. You have just learned how to tap away cravings on the spot. However, eliminating the craving may be a temporary thing. Work on the underlying fear and anger contributing to your stress. Keep making the connection and continue tapping.

Resistance to Saying No

Although you can eradicate craving in a minute or two, when faced with temptation, many people won't do it. Jimmy Durante, the famous comedian of the 1940s, used to sing, "Did you ever have the feeling that you wanted to go? And still you had the feeling that you wanted to stay? You want to go, still you want to stay. It's impossible!" Sometimes even if you desperately want to give up a compulsion, the urge may not leave. The first time Marilyn tried to tap away her desire for a cigarette, she said, "The craving is gone, but I'm gonna have it anyway!" Why wouldn't she want to forgo something she'd been moaning about being addicted to? At first Marilyn complained that she didn't have enough willpower, and here she was, after effortlessly eliminating her craving, deciding to smoke anyway.

What is this resistance all about? If you recognize yourself as a resister, tap and say, "Even though I don't want to tap to take away my craving, I completely accept myself." Use the reminder, "I don't want to." What happens? Either the resistance will melt, or you will come up with some ideas or thoughts that are blocking your success. Three common underlying beliefs that might keep you from your goal are feeling unworthy to succeed, fearing you won't be safe if you succeed, and dreading deprivation.

I Am Unworthy

Compulsive eaters have a unique problem, unlike those addicted to alcohol, drugs, and smoking. They must eat food every day to survive. Food is always on their mind. Each day they are faced with the challenge of differentiating between eating to live and the temptation to overeat in order to assuage anxiety.

The negative thoughts that plagued Laurie combined feelings of unworthiness and fear of deprivation. Before she learned Meridian Therapy, Laurie felt damned if she did and damned if she didn't. These contradictory thoughts depressed her, and led to binges.

- I deserve to die because I'm overweight.
- I will continue to be overweight, because I do not deserve to live.
- I will die unless I can eat as much as I want.
- I will die if I don't eat what I want!
- I will die because I overeat.
- If I never eat chocolate again, I might as well be dead!

I will show you how to deal with beliefs about not deserving to be healthy or free from your problems in Chapter 13, Ten Beliefs That Block Success. If you know you are stuck because you feel basically bad and unworthy, go to that chapter now. Unless you can forgive yourself and understand that your problem is an opportunity for transformation, you will remain unhappy.

Something Terrible Will Happen

Allison, Brenda, Lily, and Margaret each had unconscious fears that were so intense they couldn't stop binge eating. Each woman had trouble fighting cravings because giving up the urge to overeat meant they would lose weight, and the idea of being thin caused extreme anxiety.

Whenever Allison lost ten pounds, she immediately ate enough to gain it right back. She was apprehensive that if she became too thin, she wouldn't be able to fend off an attacker and would be injured or raped. Brenda, on the other hand, feared she would become promiscuous if she became thin. She thought her husband might leave her if she couldn't control her sexual urges. Lily grew up in the era before penicillin when people believed that a fat child was a healthy child. She feared losing her excess weight would make her vulnerable to illness. Margaret equated skinny people with those who look cadaverous as they waste away from cancer. Every time she lost weight, she imagined she must have cancer too and not know it, so she quickly gained it all back.

Perhaps as you tapped, "I don't want to," you discovered you too had some fears about safety. Irrational beliefs that are standing in your way can be transformed. Try Narrative Meridian Therapy. Talk out loud about your fear as you tap the energy points until your resistance melts.

Fear of "Never Again"

If I suggest that you pass up a cookie, cigarette, or beer or stay home from a dynamite sale, does your mind register that it means *never* having it again? Never is forever. That's a long time to be deprived of your favorite pleasure. But you can do without for one day, or even one hour. I am only suggesting that you try Meridian Therapy on your desire for the cigarette, beer, or doughnut in front of you.

Use the Five Simple Steps to confront your fear of deprivation. How do you experience deprivation? Perhaps your reminder word is simply "deprived." Or you may plaintively say, "If I don't have this one, there will never be another." It feels like this pizza, wine, or joint is the last one on earth. You may act greedy because on some primitive level you believe you won't get enough. Remember Laurie said, "If I never eat chocolate again, I might as well be dead!"

One of the principles that members of twelve-step programs learn is the *Just for Today* approach. Forever is a long time when you try to stop abusing alcohol, drugs, cigarettes, sugar, or computer chat rooms, but you can get through just one day without acting out your compulsion. It is easier to practice abstinence with Meridian Therapy. Tap as you struggle with your feelings about going without by saying, "Even though I don't want to go even one hour . . ." "Even though I can't do this . . ." or "Even though it won't work for me . . ." Be honest with yourself and don't give up.

Her Credit Cards Were Maxed Out

Arlene had been a compulsive shopper since her teen years. When she went shopping for her children's school clothes, she couldn't resist buying things for herself too. Catalogues were her passion, and she was deeply in debt. Arlene found it impossible to refrain from visiting a special boutique near her favorite spa. Each time she vacationed at the spa, she would look forward to spending money on outfits even though she had a closet full of beautiful clothes, many with the price tags still on.

She thought about not going shopping as she was getting ready to leave for a trip to the spa and felt an intense feeling of deprivation. Having recently learned how to do Meridian Therapy, she decided to try using it briefly on her ambivalence about giving up her shopping splurge. Once she was at the spa, she wasn't able to avoid the boutique. Her major triumph was buying only one dress. So Arlene decided to give tapping another chance. She began to tap about aspects of her compulsion to spend and tapped about the Super Stresses in her life.

A few months later, on her next vacation, she prepared for the trip using Meridian Therapy before she left but, again, went into the shop anyway. She felt different as she looked around and touched the fine fabrics. Tempted by the gorgeous clothing, she told the salesperson she had to think about it. Since she was determined to control her shopping addiction, Arlene tapped again and decided not to go back at all. She was jubilant. She came, she saw, but she didn't spend.

Multiple Addictions

At AA meetings people frequently drink coffee and smoke cigarettes. Overeaters also drink great amounts of coffee and diet soda and chew gum. At Debtors Anonymous meetings you will find members who are also in AA, OA, or another self-help group for addicts or compulsives. Most of the people

I counsel have switched from one addiction or compulsion to another at one time or another. Janice worked hard to become sober, but gained thirty-five pounds along the way. Marcy lost twenty-five pounds, at the same time spending all the money she had saved up for a European vacation on shopping sprees.

Giving up one behavior or substance often triggers overdoing another for two reasons. One is the feeling of deprivation, and the other is the craving cycle of the brain. When the dopamine rises and sends the message, "I gotta have it," if you are no longer drinking, smoking, spending, or eating, you will feel driven to substitute another pleasure.

The Gateway to Excess Is in the Brain

Drs. Harvey Milkman and Stanley Sunderwirth suggest in their book *Craving for Ecstasy* that human beings tend to become addicted to three kinds of feelings that produce changes in the brain's neurotransmitters: arousal, relaxation, and oblivion. In order to achieve these feelings, we use substances and behavior that affect our biochemisty.

Pleasure-seekers who enjoy the thrill of excitement look for substances or activities that give them a rush like amphetamines, caffeine, fast driving, risk taking, sky diving, or shopping. Many others enjoy the sense of contentment and relaxation that comes from eating sugar, using heroin, taking "downers," or vegging out in front of the TV. Another group looks for escape into oblivion through altered consciousness. They prefer psychedelic drugs or sleep to "go away" from their painful reality.

Giving up an addictive substance or activity is like closing your escape route. You can no longer run away from your problems into relaxation, thrill, or fantasy. The overwhelming feeling of deprivation that arises can be so uncomfortable that you may turn to another "feel-good" to take away the discomfort of withdrawal. Withdrawal is not a problem just for those abusing alcohol, drugs, or cigarettes: For example, runners also complain when they can't exercise. If you are used to medicating your stress with constant gratification, you will feel jittery and anxious when you go without your fix. The only trouble is that you simply trade in one problem for another. It is like switching deck chairs on the *Titanic*.

Achieve Sobriety

The Alcoholics Anonymous program differentiates between being "dry" and being "sober." Dry means you have stopped drinking or using drugs or activities compulsively. It does not mean you have practiced the twelve steps that will help transform your life. Sober means you are making changes in the way you live so you can cope without medicating yourself when the going gets rough. Unless you learn new ways to deal with anxiety, anger, fear, guilt, and shame, the craving cycle of the brain will continue to plague you with insatiable desires.

Choose to become conscious of the people, places, and things creating the Super Stress that triggers your binges. You can stop switching from one negative behavior to another if you practice Meridian Therapy. Tap frequently every day, whether you think you need it or not. Use the following three steps to conquer compulsion.

Conquer Compulsion in Three Steps

Recovery from compulsion is a learning process. Willpower alone doesn't work. The solution is to live life with self-awareness. What a challenge! Living a life of self-awareness means getting in touch with your feelings and becoming aware of your stress level. In other words, become an expert on you. Since you are going to be spending the rest of your life with you, stop taking yourself for granted. Keep learning from everything happy and unhappy that happens to you.

As an expert about yourself, you will need to know what you are feeling and how intensely you are feeling a particular emotion. Remember that the intense Super Stress is what causes chemical imbalances and cravings. If you aren't in touch with your emotions, how can you do anything but feel powerless when you are upset? Here is a plan to control your compulsive behavior by applying Meridian Therapy to overcome cravings.

Easy Does It

- Step one: Tune in to your cravings. Rate the intensity of "I gotta have it," on a scale of zero to ten, with ten being extreme.
- Step two: Make the connection between the urge and the stresses in your life.
- Step three: Create solutions with Meridian Therapy.

Step One

If you are serious about overcoming your urges, keep track daily of your behavior. Write it down. Make note of your binges as well as the strong urges you are able to control. Every craving is telling you something, so rate the intensity of the desire. Tap about the craving and eliminate it as it appears. Once you rid yourself of the desire you are finished. However, if you binge, write down the rating of the "I gotta have it" urgency after the fact. Then go on to steps two and three.

If you are not willing to create a daily written record of your behavior, treat yourself now before you go to step two. Say something like, "Even though I am resisting taking responsibility for my behavior, I accept myself completely." Make sure you read Chapter 13, Ten Beliefs That Block Success, for greater understanding of why you are sabotaging yourself and what to do about it.

Don't Wait for Cravings to Happen

Practice step one every day. Treat your compulsion even when you don't feel the cravings. You probably won't notice anything while you are tapping, but you are balancing the energy meridians and giving yourself a positive boost. The more you tap, the better the result will be. Some people tap in the shower or while they are in the bathroom. Tap at red lights. Be sure to always start with tapping the Karate Chop spot or rubbing the Tender spot on the chest. Tap for one or two minutes at least three times a day. You can use phrases like these:

- My compulsion
- Eating when I'm not hungry

- Drinking too much
- I can't say no to ———
- Craving for ———
- Never get over this problem
- Don't deserve to get over this problem
- Hate myself for what I do

The words may change every time you tap.

Step Two

Make the connection between your craving or binge behavior and a recent uncomfortable event. What happened in the hours or days before the binge? Some people have a continual stress, such as a job they hate. Ever-present pain can lead to daily binges. Look for your Super Stress. What situation or relationship is causing you pain?

As you write your daily log, you will begin to see patterns. Particular people, places, or things stress you again and again. You may feel powerless over many things: someone in your home who doesn't pick up his clothes, a coworker who gossips too much, a doctor who always keeps you waiting, the beloved pet who soils the rug, your child's soccer coach, the United States government, the price of gasoline, or your mother-in-law.

If you use the Daily Workout to tap away the negative emotions about the everyday events that bother you, your cravings will become less frequent because you are allowing yourself to be self-aware. Weed Whacking will help keep your stress level low. In this step look for the "over and overs," situations that continue to bother you day in and day out.

Step Three

Focus on each event or "over and over" that continues to irritate you and resolve it using Meridian Therapy. Concentrate on the underlying issues generating stress. Tap your energy points and you will release doubt and fear. As your stress is reduced, creative solutions will arise. Tap three or more times a day to erase the cravings for food, alcohol, drugs, or other compulsive behavior. Step three may take time, since the situations generating Super Stress are usually varied.

Vicki's Super Stress

Vicki's first words to me when I met her were, "I hate my job, and don't try to tell me to quit!" Vicki, a bulimic, rationalized that the pay and the hours were good even though the atmosphere and coworkers were "toxic." As she began to keep track of her binge/purges, she soon discovered that they were connected to unpleasant experiences at work. She spent a lot of time venting about her job. Tapping helped Vicki believe in herself more and more until she knew that she deserved something better. Her binge/purge behavior lessened and she eventually decided to find another job.

Human beings are complicated. There may be many aspects to your problem. When you are feeling powerless about a relationship with your spouse, memories of feeling the same way about your father may arise. Remember, Jo discovered that her cravings for juice were linked to the death of her mother when she was very young. If you aren't making progress, check out the possibility that blocking beliefs are thwarting you. Chapter 13 will instruct you in how to accomplish this. Working with a psychotherapist or joining a support group may also help you practice step three.

Learn from Every Failure

If you binge or break your resolve to "be good," feeling bad won't change things. Do a postmortem on the binge. Learn what set you off. It will help you act differently next time.

Here is how I led Vicki through the three steps when she was despondent about her out-of-control behavior.

Step One

Q: How intense was your "I gotta have it" urge on a scale of one to ten?
A: I would rate my binge an eight.

Step Two

Q: What in your life the past few days was an eight?
A: My coworker Todd ridiculed me behind my back to two others at work, and I found out. I am surrounded by idiots! I shouldn't care, because they are beneath contempt, but it hurts and I can't stop them from belittling me.

Step Three

Q: What do you want to do about this predicament?
A: I don't know. I am so angry!

Q: Are you willing to tap and see what happens?

This is what Vicki discovered as she tapped. "Todd is an asshole! I act friendly to him at work because I'm lonely. Now I am going to stop spending breaks with him or seeing him outside of work. I'll be better off talking to other people or reading a book."

This was only one episode. Vicki needed to address her relationships at work and her relationships with her family, who also belittled her. With each tapping session she felt less helpless. She became unwilling to put up with her job environment and more desirous of something better.

Use All Your Resources

Meridian Therapy will help you remove your cravings, but it may not be enough for you. Support groups, twelve-step programs, and individual counseling will also guide you toward your goal. Meridian Therapy is an excellent tool for recovery because you can use it as part of any other program for change. Along the way you may realize that you have suffered from abuse or trauma that needs to be treated by a professional. Find someone trained in the energy therapies who will welcome your participation in your own healing.

Cravings are like a red light that warns you about your

state of mind. The craving is telling you that you are overly stressed, anxious, angry, or frustrated. Don't expect to tap for a few weeks and be free of all cravings forever. Cravings will come and go throughout your life as a reflection of your emotional state. Be grateful for this built-in barometer. Pay attention, tap your troubles away whenever they arise, and compulsive urges will vanish.

chapter nine

Dissolve Panic Attacks Before They Start

Over three million people will suffer from panic disorder at some time in their lives. Chances are that you or someone close to you has been troubled with panic attacks. Anyone who has ever had a panic attack will never forget the sudden and terrifying experience. A panic attack is an occurrence of paralyzing fear and anxiety that comes out of the blue, for no apparent reason. It's like being hit with a tidal wave. You may think you are having a heart attack because you can't catch your breath. You may feel clammy, dizzy, and scared of passing out. Because these symptoms are so disturbing, you might go to the emergency room. The doctors there will reassure you that you are not in danger, but it is hard to believe you aren't about to die.

Characteristics of Panic

The National Institutes of Health lists these ten symptoms of panic attacks:

- Racing or pounding heart
- Chest pains
- Dizziness, lightheadedness, nausea
- Difficulty breathing
- Tingling or numbness in hands
- Flushes or chills
- Dreamlike sensations
- Terror, a feeling that something horrible is about to occur and you are powerless to prevent it
- Fear of losing control and doing something embarrassing
- Fear of dying

Panic attacks tend to recur over a period of months or even years. Without treatment, sufferers usually try to avoid or conceal the episodes. This can lead to problems with friends, with family, or at work. Panic attacks tend to occur randomly, so the sufferer never knows when they will happen. People with recurring panic attacks are said to have panic disorder. Recent research suggests that suicide attempts are more frequent in people with panic disorder.

Origins of Panic Attacks

Physical illness or major life stress often trigger panic attacks. Jillian was pregnant with her second child when panic attacks woke her out of deep sleep. She would walk around the house trying to get control of her anxiety, staying up for hours. She became exhausted and stressed. Jillian dreaded going to sleep because of the terror of the sudden awakening. Using Meridian Therapy, she extinguished the late-night panic attacks, and she found that tapping before going to sleep was an excellent preventative. During the day, if signs of panic arose, she simply tapped for a minute or two and nipped them in the bud.

One of the symptoms of Peter's hiatal hernia was tension in his diaphragm. When he felt it spasm, he also experienced rapid heartbeat and all the signs of a panic attack, including a horrendous fear of dying. He now taps at the first sign of distress in his body and wards off the panic. Peter is also amazed that he is now using less than half the medication he did before.

A Primitive Reaction

Panic can also be linked to our inborn "fight-or-flight" mechanism. My colleague Laura Campbell explains how the body remembers trauma and why we continue to react negatively. Here is her story:

> As a caveman was walking through the jungle, he passed a big rock, and a tiger jumped out at him. His body was equipped to deal with this emergency through a hormonal response that caused his heart to beat faster, blood vessels to constrict, and adrenaline to pump and give him the energy to fight the tiger or run. He ran back to his cave, rested for a few days and then went walking through the jungle again.
>
> What do you think happened when he saw the big rock again? His brain had saved all that information, including

sights, sounds, smells, feelings, thoughts, and physical sensations. For him the tiger was still there. It was a part of his survival instinct. Any time one of those aspects was triggered, his body, mind, and emotions would immediately respond as if back in the situation. Tapping discharges those old responses so you don't have to react to the "big rocks" in your life.

Earthquake memories

Although Eve's "fight-or-flight" reaction helped her in the Northridge earthquake, she reacted just as the primitive caveman did. Eve, a single woman, decided to go dancing one Saturday night. The dance hall had a special cushioned dance floor that gave when people walked on it. The sinking feeling and the vibrations reminded Eve of the terror of living through the earthquake in which the wall of her apartment house fell away. Suddenly she was reliving the event and went into a full-blown panic attack. She left the room and went outside, where she treated herself with Meridian Therapy. In a short while her panic was totally gone and she was able to go back inside and dance the night away.

Panic Attacks Lead to New Fears

Three problems result when someone suffers continual from panic: fear of having more attacks, fear of being crazy, and avoidance of situations that might trigger an attack. Many of those who suffer the disabling feelings of panic become consumed by the fear of having another attack. Gayle, an energetic achiever, wife, and mother, had all three problems. She was unable to go to work because she was afraid of having an attack in front of her fellow workers. Every morning she awoke to the fear. Could she make it to the office? Could she remain there all day? She was constantly monitoring her sensations to see if another panic attack was coming on.

President Franklin D. Roosevelt said, "The only thing we have to fear is fear itself." That certainly described Gayle. She was afraid she would panic when she was talking to a coworker, have a panic attack at lunch, or have to pull over while driving to work on the freeway. She had been experiencing attacks under each of these circumstances. She became tearful and worried and was unable to concentrate at her job. Her attempts to cope with her panic attacks drained her and led to extreme fatigue. Eventually the stress became so great she had to take a medical leave from her job.

When I met Gayle she was feeling miserable. She imagined she was crazy or sick. For a year, when Gayle's father had been very ill, she had juggled job, home, and infant care with long drives to help nurse him. Her responsibilities were overwhelming. Gayle was neither crazy nor ill, she was overly stressed.

She had become too frightened to drive to work on the freeway and was using side streets to go everywhere. After having a panic attack in the supermarket, she asked her husband to do the grocery shopping. Gayle developed other fears of situations she thought might bring on an attack. She became scared of driving at night or in the rain. She would no longer drive to the next town, about thirty miles away, and even with her husband driving, was afraid to go on a busy highway to visit relatives. Flying was totally out of the question. She spent most of her time avoiding any circumstances that could be risky.

Getting Well Again

As soon as Gayle learned how to use Meridian Therapy, she saw immediate improvements in her feelings and reactions. First she noticed that driving was less stressful. After three sessions of Meridian Therapy, she was able to travel on the freeway. The first time Gayle tried to drive to a neighboring town she remembered a severe panic attack she once had on that stretch of road. It triggered a terror that it would happen again. The Meridian Therapy technique put that memory to rest. She became able to remember the event without feeling any fright. Then Gayle was able to drive wherever she wanted to go.

Tapping healed the memories of other previous immobilizing attacks too. Gayle addressed each of her fears separately: worries about having an attack at work, going to the market, driving at night or in the rain, and also flying. As her irrational fears and her panic attacks disappeared, Gayle felt like a new woman.

Once Gayle felt more centered and less burdened she was able to understand that she had been operating under great stress, and this contributed to her attacks. The company she worked for was being taken over, and the threat of downsizing caused anxiety for her department. In addition, Gayle tried to do everything for her children and husband while working full time. Taking care of her own needs was low on her list of priorities. She had stopped going to the gym and was too busy to relax. As she tapped, Gayle made new decisions. She found time to nurture herself and said "No" to requests that were too time-consuming.

Once anxiety was no longer a constant companion, Gayle began to enjoy life again. She was amazed at how much energy she had spent fearing panic attacks and avoiding people, places and things that might set her off. She said, "I forgot what real life is like." The most important part of her recovery was the knowledge that she now had the power to help herself any time, anywhere by using Meridian Therapy.

If your panic attacks have been so devastating that you are on medication or being treated by a doctor or psychotherapist, you can still use Meridian Therapy to enhance your treatment.

Richard's Rapid Healing

Richard, a graduate student, developed daily panic attacks after he became engaged to Phoebe. He was insecure and worried about the relationship and about losing her love. Richard spent all his savings trying to get over his panic attacks using conventional psychotherapy. After nine months of treatment he was feeling no better. Richard had heard about Meridian Therapy and asked me to help him. He learned to use it for panic in less than thirty minutes. A week later he called to proudly inform me his panic attacks were 90 percent gone. He continued to use the tapping procedure for other problems in his life, and six months later was entirely free of panic attacks.

Five Steps to Freedom

I keep these five goals in mind when I work with people who suffer from panic attacks. You can do this too.

1. Heal the memory of the first panic attack.
2. Heal the memory of the most recent panic attack.

3. Treat panic attacks that are recurrent.

4. Address fears of future panic attacks.

5. Halt any sign of panic before it escalates.

You Never Forget

Most people can remember their first panic attack because it was so sudden and terrifying. Fred's initial experience overwhelmed him as he was driving on a crowded freeway. He thought he was having a heart attack and couldn't find a way to pull over. He later developed intense anxiety when driving near his home where the freeway expanded to five lanes. This is called agoraphobia, the fear of being in open spaces. He was so terrified of having another attack and not being able to drive across four or five lanes to safety that he began to exit before the frightening place, continuing his journey on local streets. Fred's first panic attack happened soon after his mother died. He was also having stressful job problems. He is now free of panic attacks, although he still uses tapping at times when he feels tension building as he drives.

Healing a memory of a previous panic attack means eradicating the uncomfortable feelings that arise when you recollect it. You will be able to bring the past to mind and not react. If you feel anxious, your heart races, or you have a lump in your throat as you remember what happened, it means that the memory of the panic attack is still raw, like a wound that hasn't healed. Use the Five Simple Steps as you think of that panic attack. It is essential to rate the amount of disturbance you feel right now from zero to ten as you think back. Repeat the tapping until the memory loses its emotional charge.

Your most recent attack is usually easy to recall. Lily's

most recent panic attack took place during divorce proceedings when she had to face her husband. He had severely battered her for many years before she gained the strength to leave. Now, just seeing him again terrified her. Lily used Meridian Therapy to defuse the memory of the most recent panic attack and also tapped about the abuse and danger she still felt. She dealt with her fear of having another attack at their next meeting by tapping, and was able to be in his presence a few days later without panicking.

Penny's panic attacks occurred every morning before going to work. Her panic disorder began twenty years ago when her husband was laid off from work, her marriage was in shambles and one of her children was ill. At one time she had eight or more attacks each day. Panic attacks even woke her at night. She had been on medication for ten years. When I met Penny, she was able to control much of her panic, although she still experienced some anxiety about driving and being home alone. The day after Penny learned Meridian Therapy, her morning panic attack disappeared and hasn't returned. Her other fears also abated.

Stop Holding Your Breath

Many people who suffer from panic attacks unconsciously hold their breath for a brief time. This can upset the balance of oxygen, carbon dioxide, and blood chemistry in the body and contribute to the feelings of dizziness and breathlessness. When you stimulate the energy system of the body by tapping, you will release constricted breathing. Focus on your breathing throughout the day by using the Breath Constriction Test described in Chapter 4. Breathe and rate the fullness of your breath from zero to ten, with ten being a wonderful, deep breath. Tap as you release restriction in your breathing.

You Are in Charge

Once you are familiar with the energy points and how to tap them, you can stop panic before it gets going. You might even help someone else in distress. The stress of being laid off was so upsetting that Sidney experienced an intense panic attack when he arrived home. His wife, who used Meridian Therapy for many of her problems, immediately showed him where to tap and extinguished the panic on the spot.

chapter ten

Heal Traumas and Painful Memories

Each of us has experienced at least one horrendous event in our life. When people are exposed to a terribly stressful event, they often can't get the haunting images of it out of their waking thoughts or out of their dreams at night. Anything remotely resembling that event will upset them excessively. Sometimes, an experience that only lasts a few minutes can affect you for a lifetime. These aftershocks are called post-traumatic stress disorder.

Post-traumatic stress disorder (PTSD) usually develops shortly after the traumatic event, yet symptoms may not show up for a long time. You may think that you haven't been affected by a stressful incident, but years later you can feel the symptoms of PTSD after an event reminiscent of the original trauma. Whether the traumatic incident is recent or long gone, PTSD sufferers can free themselves from the ghosts of the past by using Meridian Therapy.

How Do We Become Traumatized?

There are three types of suffering that cause lasting problems: life-threatening events, non-life-threatening but terrifying events, and severe continuing occurrences. Life-threatening happenings include natural disasters, war, physical assault, robbery, accidents, threats of harm, and terminal illness. You may also become traumatized by a broad range of distressing events such as medical or dental procedures or emergencies, fender benders, seeing your house burn down, the sudden death of a loved one, or being humiliated by a teacher in front of the class in childhood. Living in an abusive family, experiencing incest or long-term sexual abuse, withstanding domestic violence, and fighting in combat are examples of harmful continuing situations. You may be surprised to learn that even a bystander to a frightening event can be affected adversely. You could be overwhelmed just hearing about something awful happening to a loved one or seeing a disaster on TV or in a graphic film.

The Symptoms of PTSD

Kenneth didn't show any emotion when he related the horrors he had witnessed as a soldier in the Vietnam War during the Tet Offensive. He learned to numb himself by pushing the feelings away, but he still had frequent nightmares about the war. Ken found himself in his backyard with a gun in his hand, poised for action, when a rumbling earthquake struck in the middle of the night. He had no recollection of how he got there from his bed. Ellen, on the other hand, became teary when she told me about her father dying in an accident thirty years before, when she was nine.

You may react with intense anger, sadness, or fear when thinking about a terrible past event, as if reliving it. Sudden reactions, called flashbacks, may occur seemingly out of the blue and take you by surprise. Either way, there is still an open wound. You may be suffering from PTSD and not know it. With PTSD you are still living in the "there," not the "here." You continue to behave as if the event is still happening.

You suffer from Post-Traumatic Stress Disorder if:

- You keep experiencing a traumatic event through nightmares.
- You have flashbacks, feeling as if it is happening again.
- You have a severe reaction when something reminds you of the event, experiencing shaking, sweating, nausea, chills, or difficulty breathing.
- You avoid things you associate with the trauma.
- You can't remember details of what happened and feel detached.
- You are jumpy and hypervigilant.
- You have difficulty concentrating, trouble sleeping.
- You are irritable or have angry outbursts.

Perhaps you are now receiving treatment for post-traumatic stress. Check with your doctor or therapist before you try Meridian Therapy on yourself. Your therapist may already know this technique and can assist you. If not, share the technique with him.

Coping With Traumatic Events

Because traumatic experiences are overwhelming, sometimes too horrendous for the mind to encompass, victims of trauma create a number of ways to cope. Many people teach themselves to "tough it out" or downplay the impact of what has happened. They don't let on they have a problem, yet are plagued by nightmares or use alcohol or drugs. Others go into a state of denial, an unconscious way of blocking out knowledge of the terrible event. In denial we downplay the horror of the event and often say, "It wasn't that bad." Denial is a way of creating a sense of safety and security in the face of the unacceptable. Many sufferers numb their emotions and appear unaffected.

Victims may unconsciously develop a variety of behaviors to avoid any reminders of the event. They often organize their lives around not feeling any upsetting emotions. Many people won't drive on particular streets or visit places associated with their trauma. Use of alcohol and drugs is another way to deaden feelings and avoid intrusive thoughts and memories. Trauma sufferers often develop hyperalertness and startle easily. It is as if the danger is just around the corner and they have to protect themselves at all times.

Enduring childhood abuse, whether physical, sexual, or psychological, causes victims to frequently believe it was their fault. These people live a life filled with feelings of shame. They think they are basically bad or flawed and deserved the ghastly treatment received at the hands of adults. As a result many cut themselves or harm themselves compulsively. Self-inflicted pain seems to relieve the agony of the emotional pain. For some, it is a way of turning their anger toward the perpetrator on themselves.

Flashbacks Are a Fact of Life

It is difficult to go through life after a distressful event without encountering reminders that suddenly appear and cause the traumatized person to relive the experience vividly as if it were happening again. Years or even decades later, a reminder will push a PTSD sufferer into such a flashback.

Janet occasionally had flashbacks when watching movies. She suffered extreme physical brutality in childhood. Years of therapy helped her overcome most of her PTSD, yet often, when she was enjoying a movie, certain scenes triggered flashbacks. She got caught up in the memories of the past and felt emotionally distraught. After learning how to use Meridian Therapy, she tapped the energy points when the same thing happened again while she was watching a video with friends. Tapping immediately dissipated the flashbacks and allowed her to have a peaceful evening.

Paula's Story

Paula experienced a trauma when she was in her early twenties. Although she wasn't aware of it, she developed most of the reactions I have just described and suffered from PTSD symptoms for thirty years.

Paula and Gary married the summer they graduated from college and looked forward to an exciting life together. Five months later Gary became very depressed and was so distraught he found it difficult to go to work. The city was blanketed in snow and he was going to stay home due to the weather. He urged Paula to go to her job, assuring her he would be fine. As the day wore on, she worried more and more about him. When she phoned home there was no answer. She began to panic and finally decided to go home. Paula found he had committed suicide. The shock changed her whole life.

Paula was afraid that if she began to cry, she would never stop, so she didn't grieve. Instead, she numbed herself by immediately returning to her time-consuming job and acting as if nothing was wrong. Her family talked about how brave she was. Paula shut down her emotions and controlled how much she let herself cry. She lost her appetite and had trouble sleeping. The ghost of that horrendous day was always in the background.

Paula soon moved to another city to begin a new life and avoid all the reminders of the past. She later remarried and started a family. Paula stayed in denial for many years. Ten years after Gary's suicide she went to a therapist to deal with problems about her second marriage. As she told her therapist the story of Gary, she was totally unfeeling and detached from the memory. It was as if she were recounting a TV show she had seen. With the help of her counselor, Paula came to terms with Gary's suicide. She grieved and cried her unshed tears. Paula forgave herself for thinking she had contributed to Gary's death and began to feel happier.

Even so, Paula developed irrational fears. They always had to do with her second husband, Marty, not being where he was supposed to be when she phoned. Once he was at a friend's house helping to move furniture. The phone jack had become disconnected, and there was no answer. She had a panic attack and drove to the friend's house to make sure he was alive. Another time Marty called to say he didn't feel well and was coming home from work. He was more than an hour late, and she became hysterical. Paula was dialing the police as he opened the front door. This type of overreaction continued for many years.

Thirty years after Gary's death, while watching a movie in which a young widow visits the grave of her husband, Paula suddenly began to cry. The cemetery was just like the one where Gary was buried. It all came back again as if it were yesterday. As Paula cried, she realized that she couldn't remember the name of the cemetery or where he was buried. The anguish over his death had caused her to experience amnesia about many important parts of the tragic event.

By this time Paula knew how to use Meridian Therapy and was able to heal the upsetting memory at last. There are still occasional reminders that bring up moments of the original scene, but she simply taps for a minute and releases them. Paula says, "Meridian Therapy healed the very foundations of my life. The therapy I had in the past was just like pulling weeds that kept growing back. Now my life is like a beautiful green field where flowers can grow."

Veterans and PTSD

Many veterans of combat suffer from PTSD. In World War II it was called "shell shock." Vietnam veterans are still enduring the debilitating aftereffects of their experiences. Gary Craig, developer of Emotional Freedom Techniques, went to a Veterans Administration hospital and spent three days using his tapping technique with some of the patients. The results were astounding.

One veteran who had seen atrocities in Cambodia recalled a terrible incident that still upset him after over twenty years of conventional therapy. He remembered coming to a village where the Khmer Rouge had slaughtered everyone. He told of seeing blood everywhere, swollen bodies that had been decapitated, and a terrible stench. After Gary worked with him, he could recount the same event, but instead of feeling an anxiety of ten, he was at zero. "I could talk about it before, but I used to be numb. Now I am calm," he said. For many years, hundreds of memories like this had kept him from sleeping, even with medication. When he slept he had nightmares. After he learned how to tap to reduce the stress of the traumatic memories, his sleep improved and the level of disturbance remained at zero even when he tried to make himself feel upset about his wartime experiences.

You Won't Feel a Thing

Remember how Paula didn't want to let her feelings out? Many people don't want to relive the horror of a past event. There is a way to heal the pain of the past without revisiting it. Meridian Therapy is a wonderful technique to overcome traumatic memories without tears. The instructions are simple.

1. Think of a specific traumatic event.
2. Give it a title: "The time Mom pulled me by my hair," "When Bob was killed," "The rape."
3. Rate how intense your upset would be, from zero to ten, *if* you allowed yourself to relive the event in detail. **Don't try to relive it!**

4. Go through the Five Simple Steps, using the affirmation, "Even though I was raped when I was twenty, I deeply and completely accept myself," and tapping the energy points.

5. Think about how intense your upset would be, from zero to ten, *if* you allowed yourself to relive the trauma now. **Don't try to relive it!**

Repeat steps four and five until your rating is less than three. At this point you can attempt to remember the trauma in detail. Repeat this procedure until you reach zero. Test yourself by reviewing the trauma in detail. Try as hard as you can to feel upset. If there are any moments that are still disturbing, tap again.

See a Movie in Your Head

Sometimes you can't help but remember the trauma. It is like a movie playing continuously in your head. Use this approach to capitalize on what is already happening. Pretend that the memory is a video on your own home screen. When watching a video you don't have to view it from start to finish. You are able to fast-forward or rewind at will.

Chronological order is not important when treating a traumatic memory. It's OK to start with the least terrifying part of what happened. Break the story down into scenes. Go through the Five Simple Steps, tapping for each scene until you neutralize the fearfulness. Be sure to rate the level of upset each time so you can watch your response abating. When you have desensitized the worst parts, go through the memory from start to finish. Put your mental video on fast-forward and see it rapidly. Whenever there is some upset, stop and rework that scene, tapping each time. You will know you are finished when the video plays through without any emotional reaction.

What Happened to Alicia

Some traumas are too intense to try to work through in one sitting. Alicia, a college student, came to see me because she was binge eating. She told me that when she was seventeen, she had a tonsillectomy. Soon after, she had not one, but four hemorrhages in the space of a few days. Each hemorrhage was a different and terrifying experience. So much blood! She was terrified that she was dying. The hospital stopped the bleeding and sent her home three times. After the fourth hemorrhage, she was so debilitated she had to remain in the hospital. The vivid memories still haunted her. Alicia tapped to reduce the horror of each hemorrhage. In a short time she was able to recall the memory in detail without feeling any stress. When the *Super Stress* of carrying those traumatic memories was relieved, her binge eating stopped.

It Happened Over Fifty Years Ago

Yvette had been a child in Europe during World War II. Her family suffered at the hands of the Nazis and her father was sent to a labor camp. Her mother was involved with the Underground and helped the imperiled Jews. At an early age she had seen people of her village killed by the invaders. Yvette spent many years in different kinds of therapy trying to erase the aftereffects of these tragic experiences. She thought she had overcome her PTSD when an upsetting event took place in her personal life that made her feel like a powerless victim: Her home was burglarized. Suddenly she was experiencing nightmares and having flashbacks of moments of terror that had taken place over fifty years ago. When Yvette revisited the scenes of the terrifying experiences, she was able to heal her PTSD swiftly by tapping the feelings of fear, grief, and guilt as she remembered all that happened.

Stop Talking and Start Tapping

Bessel van der Kolk, M.D., an expert in the field of trauma, has shown that talk therapy is not helpful when a person is first traumatized because the part of the brain that controls verbal ability shuts down. People suffering from unresolved childhood traumas often have trouble talking about their experiences too, because that part of the brain is affected. Therefore, the best way to be treated is through a sensory or mind/body approach like Meridian Therapy.

Research with people who experienced severe stress finds that memory is stored throughout their bodies, cell tissues, and in their brain stems rather than the cerebral cortex. While experiencing deep tissue massage, I had a sudden jolt of memory about an auto accident I was involved in many years ago, when the masseuse rubbed the arm that had been sprained then.

Healing the Terror

Kristen, a twenty-eight-year-old graduate student, carried intense guilt and shame as a result of being date raped more than five years before. She couldn't concentrate and was jumpy and unhappy. As Kristen tapped, she released the misery of the memory. She worked on her fear first. Next she got in touch with her rage toward the perpetrator. Although she could remember the assault without feeling scared, she was filled with anger toward herself. Kristen blamed herself for what happened. "I should have known better," she said. Tapping helped her forgive herself and realize that she had not encouraged her date to rape her. Finally she ran the movie of the rape again from start to finish and remarked, "He is a pathetic human being." After using Meridian Therapy, Kristen's life changed for the better as she felt a new energy and strength.

My friend Grace loves living in a wooded, country area. One day, as she went out her back door, she stepped on a rattlesnake. In her panic, she started to run and fell down. The snake seemed to be chasing her. Fortunately, a member of her family heard her yell and came to the rescue. Grace was so upset she couldn't stop crying. For days she experienced intrusive thoughts about what had happened and would burst into tears over and over again. She kept replaying the scene in graphic detail. Finally Grace called me. I taught her the Five Simple Steps by phone and helped her calm down and get over her hysteria.

When her second-floor apartment was on fire in the middle of the night, and she couldn't get out, Margaret used tapping to keep from panicking. It took the firemen almost twenty minutes to rescue her. Margaret related, "During this whole incident, in which both doctors and firemen said I had only minutes to live when they got me out, I was very calm. I kept thinking, it's due to all the tapping I do for myself. Whenever I started to feel panic, I used Meridian Therapy and immediately quieted myself."

Kevin, who had also lost his home in a fire, was distraught. Tapping helped him get in touch with his despair, anger, and fear. "I'm not supposed to feel this good after what I've been through," he said. Tapping let him release his stress. His wife told him he now seemed like a different person, calm and relaxed.

The Top Five Trauma List

You may not be suffering from extreme PTSD like some of the people I have described, yet most of us have had unpleasant experiences in our lives that still bring tears to our eyes when we recall them. An easy way to heal any remaining trauma problems is to make your own "Top Five Trauma List."

You may be so used to living with the memory of the tragic death of a loved one or a terrifying car crash twenty years ago that you have buried the past and numbed the pain. Think back on your life for a few moments. What are the five most traumatic events that have happened to you in your life? Make your own private list. You don't have to share it with anyone. When you are ready, pick one of the items and use Five Simple Steps or the "You Won't Feel a Thing" variation described in this chapter. Keep tapping until you are peaceful. Remember to test whether the tapping was effective by going back to that memory and trying to feel the distress. If you do, keep tapping until it is gone.

Beverly used Meridian Therapy to come to terms with numerous traumatic memories that caused her to have a life of depression. She rejoiced, "I feel so free now. The sun has come out." Whatever your trauma, whether it happened fifty years ago or yesterday, use Meridian Therapy to rid yourself of nightmares, flashbacks, repeated thoughts, and phantoms of the past.

chapter eleven

Boost Your
Physical Health
and Well-Being

During a talk I gave to the public about Meridian Therapy, I described a case in which a colleague visited the home of a ninety-year-old woman who was recovering from pneumonia. She was terribly debilitated, had to use a walker, and needed a tank to breathe oxygen. The woman was exhausted and despondent. After a brief Meridian Therapy treatment she perked up. Her appetite improved and she started to watch TV with interest. After the second home treatment, she put away her walker and no longer needed oxygen. As I finished the story, a woman in the audience stood up and said, "That is my mother. Meridian Therapy gave her back her life."

Meridian Therapy is not intended to substitute for medical treatment. However, tapping energy points has eliminated or lessened many of the symptoms of allergies, arthritis, back pain, carpal tunnel syndrome, chronic fatigue syndrome, fibromyalgia, headaches, insomnia, multiple sclerosis, nausea, PMS, psoriasis, stomachaches, toothaches, and ulcerative colitis. The emotional aspects of physical discomfort respond quickly when you use Meridian Therapy.

Feelings About Pain

There are two elements to consider if you are using Meridian Therapy to lessen or eliminate pain or stiffness. One is obviously to tap away the pain. The other is to treat how you feel about your pain. You may be so used to living with chronic pain that you are unaware of your emotions.

Brad, a fifty-five-year-old, lived in constant pain as a result of a lifetime of back injuries and numerous surgeries. He took many medications for pain but wasn't able to relieve it. Some days the level stayed at eight and he had to grin and bear it. The first time he tried Meridian Therapy for his pain, he reduced it quickly and was delighted with the result. After that he knew he had a tool he could use as often as needed if his pain returned. Eventually he only had to treat himself once a day.

Paul lost his leg in an accident and suffered from phantom limb pain that seemed intractable. Tapping on the energy points brought up emotional feelings of inadequacy about not being a whole person. Paul continued to work with Meridian Therapy and gained a deeper appreciation of himself. He was also able to bring the pain to zero.

My Body, My Car

Your body is your vehicle. You need it to carry you through life. Unlike your car, your body cannot be traded in for a newer model. We cherish our cars and sometimes take better care of them than we do of our bodies. My car was parked in a school lot a few years ago, and while I was teaching a class, someone hit my car and drove off. The fender was dented and had to be replaced. It cost me time and money to deal with something that was not my fault! I was angry and frustrated for days. I felt as if I was being punished for something inflicted on me without my permission until I tapped away my feelings of victimization. Getting sick isn't our choice either.

Life sometimes seems unfair, sapping your time and energy as well as your pocketbook. That's how it feels when you suffer an injury or sudden illness. Perhaps your body, like your car, is getting old and doesn't have the pep it once had. Marcus was upset to discover the reason for his neck pain. One of his vertebral discs was worn thin. A sixty-eight-year-old, he didn't want to acknowledge that his body was wearing out. He resented his body for not being able to do what he wanted. His anger and sadness contributed to his pain. Meridian Therapy helped him realize that although his neck ached, he was still strong and healthy for his age and able to do many things well. Soon after, Marcus's pain subsided.

You Can Get Over It

How do you feel about your pain? Are you angry with your body for not being strong? Are you scared that, like Marcus, you are getting old and worn out? If you can't figure out how you feel about your pain, look for one of these three basic negative feelings: *mad, sad,* and *scared.* Variations of mad are resentful, annoyed, bitter, frustrated, irritated, and indignant. Sad can also be unhappy, depressed, ashamed, discouraged, disappointed, sullen, embarrassed, or useless. Maybe you are not aware you are scared but feel panicky, insecure, nervous, anxious, worried, mixed-up, or abandoned. Once you have a sense of how you feel, you can use the Five Simple Steps to ease your upset feelings. As you tap about *mad, sad* or *scared* it is possible that other aspects of your life that are bothersome will pop up. Just keep tapping until you feel neutral about all of it.

When working to ease physical pain, follow the basic Five Simple Steps. Make sure you rate the intensity of the pain before you tap. After each round of tapping notice whether the pain has diminished before you go on. Sheri reported that her menstrual cramps disappeared with this technique. Joyce was freed of a migraine headache, and Lee's arthritic thumb stopped hurting.

Stomach pains dominated Beatrice's life for five years. The middle-aged mother of three became pain-free after using Meridian Therapy. The rapid and dramatic change astounded her. She felt so healthy that it was hard to remember the distress she had endured. "It was as if the years of pain never happened, "she said.

Relieving Asthma Symptoms

Meridian Therapy is useful in eliminating many of the symptoms of asthma, such as hyperventilation, fear, wheezing, fatigue, and difficulty breathing. After leading a group through the Breath Constriction Test described in Chapter Four, I saw one of the participants, Milly, begin to smile. She had been experiencing asthmatic symptoms, and they disappeared after two rounds of tapping about her constricted breathing.

Target each symptom you are experiencing and practice the Five Simple Steps until you reach zero. You can continue to help yourself by tapping as often as possible on a daily basis. If your allergy symptoms are not responding, see your doctor for additional help.

Most asthmatics are aware of anxieties in situations or relationships that may lead to asthmatic attacks. Pearl was fearful that she would have difficulty during a forthcoming museum trip because she wouldn't be able to keep up with her tour group. She was worried that her nervousness would bring on an attack. As she tapped about her worry, she realized that the museum had elevators, and she could use them if the stairs were troublesome. After two more rounds of Meridian Therapy she was able to visualize herself enjoying the trip and feeling confident. She went on the tour without difficulty.

Alzheimer's Agony Eased

Even people with advanced Alzheimer's disease can benefit from Meridian Therapy. Most cannot tap themselves or remember the directions, but a caregiver can do it for them. Mary Sheridan, a psychotherapist who works with Alzheimer's patients, explains that she uses Meridian Therapy to soothe and calm these people when they are anxious or agitated.

"Sometimes I do the tapping for them while they are engrossed in whatever they are agitated about. If my tapping is having an adverse effect, I tap on them in my mind's eye while they are in their distress. I have about a 50 percent success rate. When it works, the person is able to leave feeling calmer and more relaxed." Mary reports that the success rate for pain is very high. Pain almost always goes away after a few rounds of tapping.

Diabetics Can Benefit

One of the most difficult challenges diabetics have is controlling their diet. I have counseled many diabetics who developed eating disorders as a result of trying to deal with the dietary deprivation demanded of them. Cravings for sugary foods disappear quickly when you tap the energy points.

June, a woman in her thirties who had been diabetic since childhood, loved fatty foods rather than sweets. Her doctor had put her on a low-fat diet due to kidney problems related to her illness. The day of her sister's wedding, June kept fantasizing about the yummy fat-laden delights that would be served. After a short stint of tapping, she was able to enjoy the celebration without stuffing herself with foods that weren't good for her.

Since Meridian Therapy takes away cravings effortlessly, there is no feeling of deprivation. You won't eat the offending food, nor will you regret it. Some diabetics become compulsive overeaters or bulimics as a reaction to the buildup of regret and loss about not being able to eat everything they want. Keep tapping and you will find it easier to stick to your eating plan.

Living with Diabetes

Diabetics never get a day off. Living with this chronic condition is hard work. Loren was wary of trying the new pump that helps manage insulin throughout the day. As a single man approaching forty, he was worried about finding love because he secretly believed that being diabetic made him unlovable and undesirable. What if women saw the bulge the pump made under his clothes? They would find out he had an illness and reject him. After using Meridian Therapy to tap away those fears and fantasies, Loren happily purchased the new technology.

Seventy-year-old Annie had already suffered eye problems as a result of diabetes. Now she was having severe circulatory problems in her feet and was terrified of having a foot amputated. She started with her fear at ten and used the Five Simple Steps. As her fear lessened, she realized in her heart that she was a strong person and could handle whatever happened in the future.

Decisions made during a traumatic event can affect you for the rest of your life. I have heard sad stories from people who developed diabetes in childhood. For some the onset was very scary and included hospitalization. Darla was one of these people. She decided that she would never have children and would die young. As a result, she unconsciously avoided intimate relationships. Meridian Therapy helped her rethink these irrational beliefs. She began to date, fell in love, and married a wonderful man.

Remembering How Much It Hurt

Jill wouldn't go to the doctor for treatment of a painful swollen wrist. Jillian, in her eighth month of pregnancy, was having panic attacks. What did both of them have in common? Each had had frightening medical experiences in the past that made her wary and afraid. When Jill was twenty, a doctor gave her a cortisone injection in her wrist without warning her how painful it might be. She never forgot that moment, and now at fifty was trying to avoid its happening again.

When Jill finally went to an orthopedist, he insisted that a cortisone injection would help. Jill asked for a couple of minutes to get ready. While the doctor was out of the room, she treated herself with Meridian Therapy. Then she calmly accepted the treatment. The shot was painful, but not as painful as she remembered, and the swelling was gone within twenty-four hours.

This was not Jillian's first pregnancy, yet she was anxious. She knew what to expect but remembered how painful delivery had been before. She used Meridian Therapy to heal the still-vivid memory of fearful moments. As she tapped, she was able to put the memories in the past. "That something happened in the past was no guarantee it would always be that way," she realized. Her panic attacks disappeared. You can use Meridian Therapy to heal hurtful or frightening memories of past medical traumas. Follow the instructions in Chapter 10: Heal Traumas and Painful Memories.

Multiple Sclerosis Benefits

MS sufferers have also reported that Meridian Therapy can ameliorate some of their symptoms. Frederika's mood lightened after she began tapping daily. She said that she was having fewer "bad" days and her attitude had shifted. Olga was so exhausted due to MS that her husband had to help her tap. She was amazed at the improvement in her energy afterward.

Psychological Factors of Illness

Whether you have diabetes, cancer, MS, fibromyalgia, or any other illness, it is important to treat the psychological aspects of your condition along with the everyday stresses of life. The physical discomfort of being sick can create depression and anxiety. You may be filled with worries about your symptoms getting worse, concerns about undergoing difficult or painful medical procedures, or fears of dying. Many people who suffer from debilitating or terminal illnesses try to take care of the feelings of their caretakers and loved ones. They may be reluctant to discuss their worries and fears with the very people who want to help them.

Your emotional state can facilitate or impair the innate ability of your body to take care of itself. Psychologist Richard Jones, Ph.D., has worked in a hospital setting for over twenty years with people who have many kinds of diseases. He tells his patients that healing is like gardening. A good gardener prepares the garden so the plants get what they need in order to grow—the right kind of soil, proper drainage, and the correct fertilizer. When given what they need, plants grow by themselves. In fact, there is such an innate drive to grow that plants have broken apart concrete sidewalks to fulfill their potential. Healthy plants have a natural resistance to most problems, but sometimes a plant becomes highly stressed and needs special attention. Meridian

Therapy will help when stress, worry, fear, or neglect have affected the state of your garden. Tap for current concerns and for those situations from the past that are still causing contamination. Allow your garden to flourish.

Caregivers Need Help, Too!

Let's not forget the people who help those who are ill or injured. Caregivers need tools for helping themselves when the going gets rough. Helping loved ones with debilitating illnesses can sap the energy of the best-intentioned people, because they are juggling two lives, their own and that of the person they care for. Caregivers can target three areas and use Meridian Therapy for each one.

1. Throughout the day perform a regular check-in for stress using the Breath Constriction Test to take the edge off worry or tension.
2. Tune in to any physical discomfort you have and use the Five Simple Steps to tap it away.
3. Notice your emotional state. Use Meridian Therapy to tap away depression, fear, anger, frustration, or sadness, whenever you need to.

Eyes Wide Open

Insomnia is rampant in our highly stressed culture. According to a recent poll of 1,014 adults conducted by the National Sleep Foundation, 56 percent experience insomnia a few nights a week or more, compared to only 27 percent in 1991. Ten to 15 percent report chronic sleep difficulties such as inadequate or poor sleep on most nights, for a month or more, compared to only 9 percent in 1991.

Having trouble falling asleep, waking in the middle of the night and being unable to go back to sleep, or waking too early are signs of insomnia. According to Dr. Gregg Jacobs, author of *Say Goodnight to Insomnia*, thoughts and behavior play the main role in perpetuating insomnia. The majority of patients who seek medical help don't have a diagnosable disorder such as depression. Insomnia often begins in response to a stressful life event such as job termination, divorce, or death of a loved one. Maybe you don't think something is bothering you because you are used to toughing it out, but insomnia may be the body's way of letting you know that something is on your mind.

Lester found himself wide awake at 3:00 A.M. with thoughts about a big project at work. He couldn't stop thinking about it. He was tense and angry. "Oh, no, I'm awake again," he thought. "Damn, now I'll never get back to sleep." Since it was cold in his bedroom and he didn't want to get out of bed, Lester used Mental Tapping as described in Chapter 3. He imagined tapping his energy points as he dealt with his negative thoughts about not getting back to sleep. Next he imagined tapping about the worrisome work assignment. As he tapped away his stress he realized that there was nothing he could do about it at 3:00 A.M., and he relaxed back into sleep.

Two Solutions for Insomnia

According to Dr. Jacobs, relaxation, letting go of tension and stress, and reframing are the answers to insomnia. Reframing means that you look at a problem from a new point of view.

Lester reframed his work anxiety by telling himself that he couldn't do anything about it in the middle of the night, and it could wait until morning. As you tap your energy points while focusing on the negative belief, new understandings will arise spontaneously. As Lester discovered, these new thoughts made sense to him and helped him see the situation in a way that felt good.

Meridian Therapy will definitely help you relax any tension you are holding in your muscles. People with "restless leg" problems have told of improvement after tapping. Use the reminder phrase "wide awake" and treat yourself to as many rounds of tapping as you need. Add the Breath Constriction Test to facilitate letting go.

Beliefs Can Keep You Awake

According to Dr. Jacobs, some of the most common negative "stoppers" are:

- I didn't sleep last night so I won't function if I don't get sleep now.
- Lack of sleep is going to make me develop health problems.
- I dread bedtime.
- Why can't I be like others and go to sleep easily?
- I can't sleep without a sleeping pill.

Keiko dreaded bedtime. Trying to get to sleep and stay asleep had become an ordeal. She couldn't remember the last time she was free of insomnia. She dreaded going to sleep and found excuses for staying up to finish last-minute chores or watch the end of a movie on TV. After using Meridian Therapy daily, she noticed a gradual improvement in her sleep. She was less resistant to going to bed, fell asleep more easily, and could put herself back to sleep without getting up if she awoke during the night. Meridian Therapy can also soothe you when nightmares suddenly wake you. Use it daily and you will tap your way to a good night's sleep without side effects or taking pills.

Allergies Respond to Tapping

Kelly was so allergic to dogs that she had built her life around avoiding them. Her new friend Ursula, a dog owner, invited Kelly to her home. Kelly explained that she couldn't go near any place a dog lived. Ursula had recently learned about Meridian Therapy and coaxed Kelly into trying an experiment. Ursula sat Kelly in her kitchen, the room with the fewest traces of her dog. She showed Kelly how to do Meridian Therapy. Kelly tapped about the worst reaction she had ever had to dogs, her fear that it would happen again, and her terror of not being able to take a deep breath if she was near dog hair. Then she took a deep breath. She could still breathe fully. There she was, sitting in a home with a dog, and she was breathing deeply! Next she risked going into Ursula's living room where the dog had been on the furniture. She had no reaction. Both women were thrilled. Now Kelly can visit Ursula free from fear.

Many people report an improvement in allergic reactions after employing Meridian Therapy. But please be sure to check with your doctor before giving up any medications for your allergies. When you use Meridian Therapy for physical ailments, you will see improvements in your attitude and in many symptoms, especially pain. There are no side effects with the tapping technique. You have nothing to lose and much to gain.

chapter twelve

Lift Yourself Higher:
The Self-Esteem Factor

When we see or hold a tiny baby, most of us feel a thrill. This new person is special and pure. Babies don't come into the world with hangups. They are born with the potential for every happiness and joy. We root for them and want them to go through life avoiding the trials we have endured. Unfortunately, many of those adorable children grow into adults who don't enjoy life because they can't value themselves or believe they are lovable.

Uncover the Past

How does this happen? Perhaps harsh parenting, traumatic incidents, or poverty corroded the golden essence you were born with. The result is lack of self-confidence and low self-worth. I like to think that as a psychotherapist I am an archeologist of the psyche. I help people uncover clues from the past to heal their present problems. When archeologists excavate a site, they bring relics covered with dirt or hardened mud out of the ground. Then workers use fine brushes to delicately wipe away the covering that has accumulated over thousands of years. Once the layers of grime are gone, the object is revealed as golden as the day it was buried.

That is what Meridian Therapy does. It helps you to gently brush away the layers of negative self-image you have acquired when life throws dirt on you. Fixing your outsides by having plastic surgery, losing weight, or driving an expensive car won't give you self-esteem. The answer is within. Your true golden nature has always been there, but you have forgotten it. Dissolve the emotional muck and reclaim your birthright by practicing Meridian Therapy.

That is what Penny did. Once she was introduced to Meridian Therapy, it took her only eight weeks to completely change her outlook on life. As she tapped, she discovered the nature of the many doubts and fears that held her back from affirming herself. She dissolved them as she tapped. "I blossomed into the happy, resourceful, content woman I am now," she declared. "I am living a great life!"

Your Emotional Standard of Living

Everyone is familiar with the phrase "standard of living" as it relates to the material things in life: what kind of car you drive or how large your house is. "Standard of living" can also pertain to your emotional level of well-being, too. When you get out of bed in the morning, you take many things about yourself for granted. For instance, you never question your name, address, or sex. What else do you take for granted? Do you dread the day because you have a "standard of living" that expects hardship and struggle, or do you rise and smile because you expect to live this day enjoying the best life has to offer?

You may not even be aware of how you set yourself up for less than the best. That was true of May, who went to her minister for counseling. She told him that she was tired of being poor. She wanted to change her "poverty conscious-ness" but didn't know how. After they had talked a while the minister reached into his pocket and pulled out a twenty-dollar bill, which he offered her. May recoiled and said, "Oh, I can't accept that." The kindly minister explained, "My point is that even when what you want is handed to you, if you have a 'poverty consciousness' you either won't recog-nize it or you won't accept it."

To raise your self-esteem, you must first become aware that you have a "poverty consciousness" about success, friends, love, work, or money. Have you ever noticed that some people always seem to have friends and enjoyable things to do, while others are lonely and believe it is hard to make friends? Some lonely people call the first group lucky and call themselves unlucky. People with low self-esteem think they don't deserve to have the happiness and peace of mind others seem to have. These beliefs can become self-fulfilling prophecies. Therefore, those with negative self-images settle for jobs and love relationships that are unfulfilling. They affirm that they aren't as exciting or good-looking as others, so they should be content with their lot.

Carmen's Tale of Woe

Carmen was fed up with her unfulfilled life. She was frustrated because she kept comparing herself to others and felt like an outsider. "It's not fair! Other people have happiness come easily. They are better looking, thinner, and have more fun," she said. " I never get anything. Why, even when I was a child and played princess with my best friend, I was always the servant and she got to be the princess." After many years of being told she wasn't worthy by her mother and being put down by her few friends, Carmen couldn't visualize herself having more in life.

Carmen described her childhood as cold. Her parents acted cold. Even their house was kept uncomfortably cold! As a very young child, Carmen learned to make others feel good and became adept at taking care of herself when no one else did. She learned to go to neighbors' homes where people welcomed her and gave the sweet little girl tasty snacks. She laughed and had fun with them. Carmen figured out how to be nice to herself by hoarding pennies to buy ice cream, a treat she rarely got.

Using Meridian Therapy to heal her unhappy memories, Carmen was able to value her resourcefulness instead of blaming herself for past actions. She began to speak up and assert herself with others and was pleasantly surprised at the changes in her life now that she likes herself more.

Rich or Poor?

What is your standard of living? Do you consider yourself rich or poor? Are you a new-car or a used-car person?

Do you stay within the comfort zone of "less than" that you have created? Some students create a niche when they think of themselves as maintaining a "solid B" average. Athletes do the same thing. When sports enthusiasts converse they often label themselves. Ryan, a golfer, says, "I shoot in the low nineties." Bowlers also rate themselves by their performance averages, as do baseball players. If you are ready to move beyond your limitations, take this challenge.

The Comfort Zone Challenge

Decide where in your life you are stopping yourself from having it all: income, housing, sports achievement, grades, romance, job, or another area.

Start with one of these affirmations or make up your own. Then proceed to tap the remaining energy points.

- Even though I stop myself from achieving _____. I deeply and completely accept myself.
- Even though earning _____ dollars seems beyond me, I am a good person.
- Even though I can't do better because it would require too much of me, and might hurt those I love, I profoundly love and accept myself.
- Even though I am afraid to challenge my "standard of living" because I might find out I am truly inadequate, God loves me.

Self-Destructive Thoughts

You may discover that many so-called minor negatives can pile up and create a major emotional blockage that hinders your growth. Nick persisted in using Meridian Therapy to change his outlook on life. He says, "I find myself still performing many tapping processes every day. I sigh a lot. And with each sigh I smile and take an even deeper breath to help that sigh do its work."

Here is how Prudence helped herself. She summed up her negative view of herself in one sentence and affirmed, "Even though I am worthless, superficial, uninteresting, unattractive, stupid, and everyone knows it, I completely and profoundly accept myself." Then she tapped the energy points over and over again. After a while her words seemed absurd to her. Like Prudence, most of us judge ourselves by what we don't achieve and who we have come to believe we are. Negative thoughts intrude in our waking life and even in dreams. We are both judge and jury and condemn ourselves to a lifetime of punishment in a jail of our own making.

Five Killer Beliefs

Giving power to any or all of these thoughts will erode your view of yourself and limit your happiness. Are you guilty of believing these are true?

- I am worthless.
- I don't deserve to be happy.

- I don't like myself.
- I don't love myself.
- I am not a good person.

Randy's Surprise

Randy didn't even know he had imprisoned himself in false belief until he was confronted with a dilemma. Randy and his sister Rona had a distant relationship that was cordial but not close. They lived in different states and rarely saw each other. One Christmas when the whole family was together, Rona confided that she wanted to heal the rift in their relationship. She asked Randy to have lunch with her the next day.

The next morning Randy was unhappy. He agreed to go with Rona, but he really didn't want to. "I am not interested in getting close to her," he told his wife. "I have tried before, but it never works out." Should he be true to himself or force himself to go to please his sister and the family? Randy had used Meridian Therapy before for other problems and was surprised when his wife suggested that he tap about his ambivalence.

After two rounds of tapping he suddenly began to sob. "I hate myself," he cried. He kept tapping and exclaimed, "Now I understand it all." To this day Randy's wife doesn't know what happened. All she knows is that he went out with his sister and had a wonderful time. He came back with new respect for her. A few days later he told his wife that his body felt different as well as his energy. His outlook about his whole life had changed. "I feel confident that I can be successful in whatever I want to do," he declared.

Get Out of Jail Free

As children most of us played Monopoly. The "get out of jail free" card was a prize. If you landed in jail, you didn't have to languish or pay a penalty. If you had the card, you could get out immediately. What kind of sentence have you pronounced for yourself? Are you condemned to be unloved, poor, unhappy, or sick? You can get out of jail any time you want by targeting any or all of the Five Killer Beliefs. Practice Meridian Therapy until you know that you deserve good things, you are valuable and lovable.

What's Your Secret?

Jamie, a former fashion model, told me that when she was getting started in her career she was very nervous about going out in front of an audience at fashion shows. A more experienced model gave her a tip. She told Jamie to look at herself in the mirror and think, "I've got a secret." Then walk out on the runway radiating that thought. What was Jamie's secret? "I'm great and I know it!"

You have a secret too, but you may not be aware of what it is. Perhaps you have a talent or skill that others admire but you minimize. I believe that each of us is born with a gift. That gift is something we can be or do without any effort. Because it is so easy, we tell ourselves it doesn't count, even when others ooh and aah at our achievements. I marvel at people who can play a musical instrument by ear or fix things without reading the instructions. Maybe your talent is in organizing things, being physically coordinated in sports, having a knack for decorating, or being highly intuitive.

The twelve-step programs often urge members to "act as if" something were true. If you don't believe in yourself, try this strategy. Make a name tag to pin on your clothing. In dark ink print these letters: IALAC. They stand for *I am lovable and capable*. Wear this sign for a week and remind yourself that this is your secret. See what happens.

Self-Discounting Beliefs

Hardcore self-critics won't want to admit they are worthy of love and praise. The great comedian Groucho Marx once wrote this to a country club: "Please accept my resignation. I don't care to belong to any club that will accept me as a member." Stop resigning from opportunities in your life. Here are six common beliefs that are guaranteed to make you miserable.

- I'm not capable.
- I am ugly.
- I am stupid.
- I have no skills.
- I have no talents.
- I'm not good at _____ (talking to people, cooking, saving money, finding love, saying "No," and so forth)

Many people call themselves stupid or untalented because they have an unrealistic standard they are comparing themselves to. How do you know that you are stupid or incapable?

Where is the evidence? Did an unloving parent or sibling label you? Create a long list of all the things you are not good at. Write "I am not good at saving money compared to my brother," or, "I am not good at mixing with strangers at parties compared to my friend Bobby." Use the Five Simple Steps for each one. If you don't have a reality check, you will never be good enough to please the irrational inner critic.

Indentured for Life

Susanna, a thirty-seven-year-old single woman, had both an inner critic and an outer critic in the form of her mother. When she went back to school to finish her education, Susanna began to have trouble studying. If she didn't do her homework, she was too embarrassed to go to class because she had to be perfectly prepared, or else! Susanna discounted herself all the time because she wasn't able to live up to her self-imposed, impossibly high standards.

When Susanna used Meridian Therapy to lessen her fears of being imperfect, she realized that by believing she was stupid or unskilled she was accommodating her critical mother in order to stay in mother's good graces. After a lifetime of being disparaged, she had very little self-confidence, and she was exhausted striving for perfection. Perfection meant living up to her mother's expectations. These requirements could change at her mother's whim, so Susanna could never hope to reach her goal. She was in bondage to her mother. Susanna thought of herself as incompetent and depended on mother for financial support and approval. When her mother withheld praise, she felt even more unfit. She might as well give up and drop out of school.

Tapping helped her put the situation into perspective. Susanna was able to realize that she was now an adult and no longer had to obey her mother's commands. She was free to disagree with mother's standards. Besides, slavery was abolished over one hundred years ago! Since then Susanna has been enjoying school and is delighted with her good grades.

Ducks or Swans?

Most of us have heard the story of "The Ugly Duckling" in childhood. The poor little "ugly" one was picked on by the other ducklings and made to feel stupid and awkward. Then one day he saw some wondrous creatures swimming in the pond. When he looked at his reflection in the water, to his amazement, he discovered that he looked just like the graceful swans. No wonder he had so much trouble trying to be a duck. He was really a swan. Once he knew that, he was able to join the other swans and be his true self.

What Susanna didn't realize was that she was born into a family of ducks and she was a swan! The ducks demanded that she conform to their criteria. She had to squelch her natural talents and curiosity in order to fit in and please others. Susanna didn't know she was a swan. The more she tried to be a duck, the more she felt like an outsider or someone who was simply born permanently flawed. Each time Susanna used Meridian Therapy, she got more and more in touch with her true swan nature. As she began to trust her own values, she felt less stressed and more powerful.

Banish Limiting Beliefs

Refer to the six self-discounting beliefs or make up your own. Expand them in your own words. "I'm not capable" might become "I'm not capable of taking care of my checkbook," or, "I'm not capable of being in an intimate relationship." Perhaps you'll create a special list of all the things you don't think you are capable of. Use Meridian Therapy to explore each one. As positive thoughts arise, write them down next to the negative ones. When you are finished, test yourself by speaking each negative idea out loud in a strong voice. Is it still true?

Do this with each idea that tears down your self-image. When you tell yourself, "I have no skills," which skills are you missing and in what areas of your life? Are you deficient in computer skills, driving ability, knowing how to play tennis, or cooking? Be as specific as you can. Tap each opinion until change occurs.

I believe that you deserve the very best, and you deserve to believe it too. If you are committed to improving your self-esteem, use the Daily Workout. A few minutes of tapping a day will make a permanent difference in your life.

Part Three

Troubleshooting: Getting Back on Track with Meridian Therapy

chapter thirteen

Ten Beliefs That Block Success

Have you ever tried and tried to solve a problem or get over a bad habit, but nothing you did worked? Often when the frustration increased, you gave up. Perhaps there is a reason you aren't making headway. A negative core belief may be stopping you. We all have core beliefs, powerful thoughts rooted deep in our unconscious minds. Core beliefs are like hidden computer programs that are beyond our conscious awareness, yet they shape our behavior. They can be positive or negative.

Programmed by the Past

Core beliefs usually arise in childhood from pronouncements or casual remarks by adults who taught you manners and morals. Since you assumed that Mom, Dad, the teacher, or the minister was always right, whatever they said must be the truth. These real or imagined statements became embedded in your belief system as if they were commandments.

Many of our beliefs are really only the convictions of authority figures in our past, and we don't realize it because we were "brainwashed" to go along with what we were taught. Right now many of these tenets feel true; maybe you learned that they are unquestionable. Positive beliefs have the power to create; negative beliefs destroy. If in living by their so-called truths you are harmed more than helped, perhaps they're not the whole truth.

Common Core Beliefs

Here are ten familiar negative core beliefs that may block your path to health and peace of mind. Identify which declarations strike a chord as you read the following list.

- I don't deserve to get over this problem.
- God is punishing me.
- I will never get over this problem.
- I'm not sure I want to get over this problem.
- If I get over this problem I will lose my identity.
- If I get over this problem it will be bad for someone else.
- If solve this problem I will be deprived.
- If I get over this problem I won't be safe.

- There are some good things about having
  this problem.
- It is impossible to get over this problem.

Now is the time to tap away destructive core beliefs. When a belief harms you more than helps you, and you still aren't willing to let it go, tap about your unwillingness. Start with the affirmation, "Even though this belief is hurting more than helping me, and I want to continue to make my life miserable anyway, I totally forgive myself and deeply accept myself." Tap until you no longer want to make yourself miserable.

Some people don't want to give up their negative beliefs even though their lives are made unhappy by holding on to them. If you are one of those people, take a piece of paper and make two columns. Write the negative belief on the top. Title one column "How It Helps Me," and the other, "How It Harms Me." Under each column list the ways this idea adds to your life or makes your life uncomfortable or unbearable. When you are finished, read over your lists and decide which influences your life more, help or harm.

If you aren't sure whether you are hindered by negative core beliefs, the stories that follow may help you identify any thoughts that are sabotaging your success.

I Don't Deserve to Get Over This Problem

Feeling unworthy will lead you to act in ways that undermine your goals. Your head may tell you that you are OK, but a small place deep within denies it. Some people actually hear a voice, usually Mom or Dad, that tells them they are unlovable, a loser, stupid, and will never amount to anything. No matter how much you fight that voice, it keeps coming back.

I Don't Accept Myself

Colleen is a successful self-employed consultant who desperately wanted to be free of her anxiety problem. Whenever she said the affirmation, "I deeply and completely accept myself," she began to sob. "I can't accept myself. I am bad and don't deserve to get better," Colleen maintained.

Her "I don't deserve" attitude influenced many areas of her life. As long as she was sure she was undeserving, she wouldn't allow herself to feel happy. When she challenged the "I don't deserve" by tapping, it brought forth many memories of an abused childhood during which Colleen decided she was bad and unlovable. Meridian Therapy helped her heal the pain of these memories and see herself in a new light of self-acceptance.

I Have to Suffer

A poet named Cesar wanted to overcome his stage fright. He was often called upon to read his poetry in public. It was an ordeal. As he tapped, he understood that performance anxiety was a long-time companion. The dread was so familiar it was hard to imagine being without it. In fact, if he wasn't scared, he might even enjoy his performances, and that wasn't allowed! "I guess I'm not supposed to feel happy. To my way of thinking, life consists of burdensome things that I have to get through," he explained. Somehow he had created a view of life as a very hard journey, one he could get through, but only with great effort and little joy.

If you identify with Cesar, ask yourself what you are afraid would happen if you let yourself be happy. The first response will be "Nothing. Why wouldn't I want to be happy?" Keep asking yourself and notice what other thoughts arise. If you aren't sure this is a blocking belief, use Meridian Therapy with the phrase "I don't deserve to be happy." You may realize you already know why you aren't supposed to feel worthy, but you haven't wanted to acknowledge that you know.

Never Good Enough

Becky was frustrated because she wasn't having the success she wanted at losing weight. Each time she lost a few pounds she would binge and regain them. She was angry with herself. Becky was a typical "good girl," always taking care of her family and never expressing her own feelings or asking for what she wanted. "When is it my turn? When do I get what I deserve?" she raged. Then she started to cry as she realized she secretly believed "I'm not lovable. I'm a disappointment."

Whatever Becky did was never enough, according to her mother. She decided early in life that maybe she was born bad and there was something inherently wrong with her. People like her weren't supposed to be successful. Becky wasn't even conscious of the ways she made her negative beliefs come true until she used Meridian Therapy. As she tapped she was able to affirm that she had always been enough. She now knew that it was OK to succeed at whatever she chose, and she chose to lose weight.

God Is Punishing Me

"God is punishing me," said Vanessa, who believed that smoking was a form of gluttony, a sin. She told herself that

God had forgiven her so many times, maybe HE was fed up with her. I asked her if the "three strikes you're out" rule also applied to sinning. Since she had decided what God's rules were, she was punishing herself because she knew God would definitely want to chastise her. Although her conscious mind thought that God was Love, her unconscious feared God's wrath.

Most of my clients have a strong faith in God or a Higher Power, yet in their lives they act as if they are the servants of a disapproving God. Which would you rather be? The first step in Vanessa's transformation was to forgive herself for not being perfect. Meridian Therapy helped her stop fearing God's vengeance. Tapping restored her faith in a loving and forgiving God and in herself as a child of God. She let go of second-guessing the deity's wishes for her and succeeded in overcoming her compulsion.

I Will Never Get Over This Problem

If you have a problem or fear that has lasted for many years, perhaps your whole life, you may have resigned yourself to live with it. You may have tried many ways to overcome a fear, addiction, anger problem, panic attacks, or a persistent bad habit. "What if I fail again? What will people think?" you ask yourself. Then you predict the worst-case scenario. The embarrassment keeps you from trying something new, so you just give up.

Marlene's panic attacks had been a part of her life for so long that she doubted she would ever be free of them. They started after the birth of her first child more than five years ago. Medication helped somewhat, but she still experienced lightheadedness and hyperventilation occasionally. She was wary about trying Meridian Therapy because it seemed radical and unusual compared to the treatment she had had in the past. First she tapped her distrust that Meridian Therapy could work for her. Next she tapped her negative attitude, that she would never be free from anxiety. The panic attacks ended after she used Meridian Therapy

No Rest for the Weary

Donna discovered that her sleep problem had many aspects. After discovering that she was molested by a neighbor as a child and healing the memory using Meridian Therapy, she was able to sleep better, but she still wasn't getting a good night's rest. Sleep deprivation took a heavy toll on her outlook. She believed that she would never be over her difficulty.

Going through a divorce and worrying about how the outcome would affect her children added to her tiredness. Then her ex-husband, who suffered from depression, had a relapse. Donna's anxiety escalated. She was afraid that she would also break down, and then what would happen to her children?

Practicing Meridian Therapy, Donna discovered other aspects from her past that contributed to her growing fear. She remembered a time when she was in college and had to get medication for her anxiety and depressed mood. As she tapped she thought, "There's a big cloud looming over my family." Donna's grandmother, mother, and sister all had suffered from bouts of depression. "I'm next," she agonized. Further tapping produced this conclusion: "My mother and sister had trouble sleeping when they were depressed. I don't want to be like them."

Donna began to feel better after she discovered the roots of her anxiety and discharged the fear. She stopped worrying as she realized that her ex-husband's situation wasn't permanent. He could get treatment and feel better soon. She made decisions about lightening her load of responsibility for the family. Other relatives could assist. She could see the light at the end of the tunnel and her sleep improved.

I'm Not Sure I Want to Get Over This Problem

You may be asking yourself why anyone would want to hang on to a problem that is causing grief and pain, yet many people do. On an unconscious level they expect a payoff to the problem, some reward that makes the suffering worthwhile.

Joe, a man in his late forties, felt lonely and alone. He saw families with happy parents and playful children, but he had no one to love. He was angry at the world. Through Meridian Therapy, he learned that keeping the feeling of anger alive let him hold terror at bay. As he tapped, he made a startling discovery. His belief was, "If I get over this problem I will die." You see, Joe believed that if he gave up his anger problem and had nothing to distract him, he would discover that life was meaningless. Therefore he had no reason to live and might as well commit suicide.

Joe was suffering from depression, which caused him to see existence as dark and miserable. Once he received treatment for his condition he was able to see the world from a new perspective. Tapping daily also helped. If you think you might be hanging on to a problem because there is something even worse waiting for you, please see a trained professional. Meanwhile, you can use Meridian Therapy and observe what you think or feel.

Self-Defeating Payoffs

Here are some other payoffs to holding on to painful problems. You can use Meridian Therapy for any one of the following self-defeating thoughts or focus on "I'm not sure I want to get over this problem."

- Others will make it up to me because they'll feel upset or guilty.
- People will feel sorry for me.
- I can avoid taking responsibility for what I do, say, or feel.
- I'll have an excuse for poor performance.
- I can keep a distance from others and avoid relationship problems.
- I get to share and feel close to others who have the same problem.
- I feel a sense of intensity and feel more alive.

If I Get Over This Problem I Will Lose My Identity

Carolyn Myss, the well-known medical intuitive, challenges us to stop labeling ourselves by our wounds. Many people identify themselves as addicts, children of divorce, victims of abuse, or compulsive personalities. It becomes part their personality. She calls that "woundology." Who will you be if you are free of your traumatic memories, your panic attacks, your compulsions, or your migraines?

Amanda's Challenge

Amanda, an extremely bright and talented woman, was working at a job far below her capabilities. She was miserable. Although the workplace atmosphere was negative, and there were few chances for advancement, she felt loyal to the company. She wanted to leave, yet kept rationalizing that she might not get another job in a difficult market, and it wasn't nice to quit.

Tapping helped her understand that the turmoil created by her job was like an old friend. Amanda's whole life had been filled with turmoil. She came from a large family of dysfunctional people. As the oldest, she often took over as a mother figure for her younger siblings. She remembered holding the family together.

If she gave this up, what would replace it? Who would she be? She was used to coping with disordered and difficult situations since childhood. Her motto might be "What's wrong? Nothing's wrong; that's what's wrong." Meridian Therapy enabled Amanda to rid herself of her need to suffer. Finally, the day came when she knew she was ready for a job in which she would feel happy, and she quit.

What's Your Emotional Standard of Living?

Your identity is also influenced by your *emotional standard of living*. How much happiness or success you allow yourself to have is similar to how much money you think you are capable of earning. Do you have an imaginary ceiling you think you can't go above? Jennifer discovered that her fear of flying was linked to her limited sense of herself.

Jennifer, a talented psychologist, wasn't sure she wanted

to give up her intense fear of flying. She convinced herself that she didn't like travel and had no wish to visit faraway places. She saw herself as a homebody. She was known and respected in her community, where she practiced and taught. If she gave up her fear of flying, she wouldn't have an excuse to turn down opportunities to travel and make presentations before large audiences. Being a big fish in a little pond was comfortable. What if she wasn't good enough to compete in a larger marketplace? She challenged her belief that she wasn't good enough and tapped it away. She soon decided she could handle a new lifestyle and was free to choose if or when she wanted to travel. Before long she was invited to do presentations in another country and happily flew to her destination.

If I Get Over This Problem It Will Be Bad for Someone Else

Can you really harm another by leaving your problems behind? Some people think so. Bobbie didn't know that this core belief was at the heart of her relationship problem. Bobbie kept choosing the wrong man to love. She was attracted to men who had major problems, sometimes addicts, often "losers," and she had spent many years in therapy questioning her self-esteem and inability to find the right relationship.

Because she wasn't sure which of the ten negative beliefs were at work in her unhappy love life, she decided to tap each one. As she tapped "If I get over this problem, it will be bad for someone else," she thought about how her mother had always commiserated with Bobbie. It was her mother who ran to her rescue when she was left alone and penniless after an unhappy marriage. She next remembered the time her sister revealed that Mother thought of Bobbie as her "unlucky child." Bobbie was upset because she didn't think of herself as unlucky.

The pieces started coming together as she continued using the Five Simple Steps. She knew her mother needed to be needed, and she was obviously pleasing mother by continuing to need Mom's emotional and financial support. If she stopped being unlucky in love, her mother wouldn't be needed anymore and might become unhappy. Bobbie would be to blame. All of this was happening on an unconscious level. Once Bobbie discovered her negative collusion, tapping helped her change her attitude. She was able to stop being part of a game that was really hurting her, not her mother.

Emotional Blackmail

A relationship in which someone gives up happiness and independence in order to make another person happy or secure is not healthy. If someone you hold dear remains miserable, no matter how hard you try to please, you may feel guilty. You are supposed to know how to take care of the one you love, but they keep changing the rules. I call it emotional blackmail. Once you know that no one can make you happy except yourself, you will be free to stop trying to satisfy another.

If you believe it will be bad for someone else if you get over a problem, think about the situation. Use the Narrative approach. Tap as you talk out loud to yourself about what will happen when things change. Keep this up until your attitude changes.

If I Solve This Problem, I Will Be Deprived

During a demonstration, using Meridian Therapy to overcome cravings, I asked for a volunteer who loved chocolate. Gus stood up. I gave him a piece of Belgian chocolate and asked him to smell it and taste it to increase his desire. A few rounds later, he said he liked chocolate but didn't really want to eat that piece now. He could "take it or leave it."

Before he went back to his seat, however, he anxiously asked, "Can I undo it later?" Gus was distraught because he didn't expect to lose his craving *so fast*. His fear was that he would now hate chocolate and not want to eat it *ever again*. I explained that he always has free will to choose what to do or not do. Meridian Therapy doesn't turn you into a zombie. At that moment he could have eaten the rich chocolate, but he didn't really want to. He didn't feel deprived when he threw the candy away, yet after years of feeling guilty about indulging in chocolate, Gus wasn't able to conceive that freedom to say *no* doesn't feel like deprivation.

Overcome the Pain of Loss

You may be one of the millions of people who are compulsively drawn to pleasurable activities and substances as a way of feeling good when you are feeling bad. Taking away the cigarettes, candy, pizza, alcohol, or drugs may leave you vulnerable to underlying feelings of fear, anger, or depression. If you are a slave to your compulsion, you can't know what it feels like to be free of that bondage. You may imagine you will feel bereft and disconsolate. Life will be dull and meaningless. You will have nothing to look forward to.

The opposite is true, but you are afraid to find out. Tapping away a craving will leave you with a feeling of well-being. No one is coercing you. There is no outside pressure or guilt trip being forced on you. You will just lose interest in the object of your desire. If this upsets you, please tap immediately on the idea that you will feel deprived and miserable. If you are still fearful that you are going to have to forgo pleasure forever, use Meridian Therapy with the reminder phrase "This craving, just for today." Only after you come to terms with the negative belief can you allow yourself to deal with your cravings. Then you can follow the instructions in Chapter 8 about conquering cravings and compulsions.

You Can't Make Me Do It

Angela experienced the fear of deprivation in a different way. Her goals were to stop smoking, cut back on sugar, and exercise more. She enjoyed martial arts and went to class, but didn't want to buckle down and do what was necessary to advance to a black belt. In fact, Angela didn't want to do anything she labeled "unpleasant." In her mind, forcing herself to spend time practicing or studying karate felt like punishment. Anything that would take time away from feeling the pleasure of eating and smoking made her anxious.

Angela knew that she was rebelling against the harsh and rigid parenting of her childhood, when she was not allowed to have fun playing with her friends and had to obey the punitive rules set down by her unloving parents. Until she began to use the tapping process, she couldn't control her intense rebellious feelings and "I'll show you!" actions, which continued to sabotage her best efforts. Angela tapped every day to deal with her irrational feeling of deprivation. Soon she began to exercise more, stopped smoking, and was eating a healthy diet because she wanted to.

If I Get Over This Problem, I Won't Be Safe

Edith wanted desperately to lose weight, but began having panic attacks when she lost ten pounds. She was puzzled because she truly desired to look slimmer. On the list of blocking beliefs, the possibility that she wouldn't be safe if she lost weight hit home. On an unconscious level she was terrified of being smaller. Edith was molested by her father from the time she was three until she was thirteen. She couldn't fight him off, and nobody rescued her. Edith feared that smaller meant weaker. Someone larger than she was could physically overwhelm her and hurt her, and she wouldn't be able to fight back. Meridian Therapy helped eliminate the frightening core belief and allowed her to shed pounds without panic.

Trina Was Tough

There was no doubt in Trina's mind that she could take care of herself. "I can stand up for myself against everyone," she said, and she did! Yet Trina wondered why her boss cringed when she said she wanted to talk to him. She was unaware that her aggressive manner put him off. Sometimes when she became enraged she lost friends because of her hostility. Trina hoped Meridian Therapy could help her become less abrasive.

Tapping uncovered the source of Trina's problem. She was severely beaten as a child, feeling totally powerless in the face of her mother's overwhelming fury. She had to be strong in order to survive. "I keep the rage to scare people so they don't hurt me, " she said. "I am afraid to give up my aggressiveness because I will be powerless and alone."

Trina used Meridian Therapy to deal with memories of her abused childhood. She remembered her mother saying, "Don't you defend yourself or I'll give you more!" As she healed she was able to become softer and more vulnerable and still feel safe.

Can I Ever Trust Again?

Many women who have been sexually abused in childhood experience problems in intimate love relationships. Crystal wanted to feel close to her boyfriend, Burt, but when he moved in with her, she found herself pulling away or feeling anger toward him. When she let herself be close she felt unsafe. Referring to the traumatic experiences of her childhood, she thought, "I died when I was a child. I built a wall around my heart. If it comes down I'll die." Healing the wounds of the past takes time. As Crystal used Meridian Therapy, she began to feel safer with Burt and was able to enjoy being intimate with him.

There Are Some Good Things About Having This Problem

Jeri's finances were chaotic. Paying bills was like Russian Roulette because she didn't balance her checkbook. "I live in a state of anxiety every day," she affirmed. Imagine Jeri's embarrassment when she tapped about her frustration and discovered that deep down she didn't want to manage her money. As long as she didn't let herself know how much money there was, she could spend recklessly and hope for the best when the bills arrived.

"My spending lifts me out of my negative emotions," Jeri said. Compulsive shopping allowed her to feel pleasure and maintain a state of denial about the pain of her life. Jeri's ex-husband was in danger of losing his job. If he stopped helping out, she would have to take on more financial responsibility to support her children.

Grownups know how to balance their checkbooks and budget. Grownups take responsibility for their actions. As long as she didn't act like an adult, Jeri could stay a child. Children get taken care of and bailed out by kind friends and relatives.

When her anxiety became overwhelming, Jeri used Meridian Therapy to address the turmoil. The first thought that surprised her was, "If I don't have chaos I will have to be mature and responsible like my parents. Oh, no, I'll turn into my parents!" Jeri dealt with that fear by tapping. As she honored the capable adult part of herself she stopped letting the angry, helpless child within run her life. She opened a brand-new checking account and started from scratch. Jeri also decided to find new ways to increase her income.

It Is Impossible to Get Over This Problem

When you tell yourself, "I will never get over this problem," it means you believe there is a solution, but you have given up hope of finding it. "It is impossible to get over this problem" means you think there is no solution to your problem. Not even a miracle can help you. Two blocking beliefs stood in the way of Damon's healing: "I don't deserve to get over this problem" and "It is impossible to get over this problem."

"What he did to me is permanent and can't be changed. I am damaged," is how forty-five-year-old Damon described himself as he came to terms with a terrible memory. Damon had been molested as a small boy by a man he trusted. As a result, all his life he had felt different from others, ugly, misunderstood, angry, and sad. Despite his many talents and great intelligence, he thought of himself as a failure. Damon secretly believed that he was to blame for the traumatic incident. He was filled with self-loathing about all the bad things he had done in his life since then and the people he had harmed through his rage and lies. "I've ruined my life. What I have done to my family is unforgivable."

Damon saw himself as someone condemned to be miserable for the rest of his life, since he believed that the damage inflicted when he was eight was impossible to heal. Damon first felt fearful and angry when he tapped his energy points. After two or three rounds he said, "I'm just a human being, and they mess up a lot. I've tried to make good come out the unforgivable things I did." More tapping led him to understand: "The root of the whole thing is what was inflicted upon a little kid who couldn't possibly cope with it. The important thing is to learn from it and go on." Damon tapped about the self-blame after the molestation. "It's going to be OK, and I'm OK," he said. About the perpetrator, Damon explained with compassion, "He was a troubled person who didn't know the right way to deal with children." Once Damon was free from his paralyzing belief, he began to like himself more and felt more power over his life.

With Meridian Therapy, the stumbling blocks of negative core beliefs that hold you back can be uncovered and demolished. The ten blocking beliefs aren't true and never were. As you tap you will know the truth, and the truth will set you free.

chapter fourteen

When Meridian Therapy Doesn't Work

You may have turned to this chapter because, after following all the instructions about performing Meridian Therapy, you are not experiencing results. Troubleshooting is called for. There can be many reasons why the technique doesn't seem to be working. Let's explore what could be happening and what to do to achieve success.

You Don't Notice a Change

Positive transformations that result from using Meridian Therapy often feel so "normal" that you may not even be aware of them. Toby sounded morose when I talked to him during his fourth session. He described feeling depressed and withdrawn. He reported that he doubted the efficacy of Meridian Therapy. During our conversation he mentioned that his wife reported that he sometimes woke up singing the morning after a

Meridian Therapy session. Toby couldn't remember that happening but trusted that she hadn't made it up.

Erin felt anxious when making love with her husband because she needed constant reassurance that he loved her. She held back and didn't allow herself to fully enjoy the pleasure of being close to him. She tapped about this during a few Meridian Therapy sessions but didn't report feeling anything shift. Two or three months later, her husband asked her if she was still obsessed with doubting his love for her, and she realized that the distress was no longer there.

Toby and Erin's lives are like intricate tapestries filled with many motifs, colors, and textures. After using Meridian Therapy they were not aware of major changes, but others began to notice the alterations taking place. Sometimes if you don't think you are making headway with Meridian Therapy, ask your friends, coworkers, or loved ones to give you feedback. Keeping a diary is another way to help yourself measure the changes.

Check Your Technique

When your negative emotions don't fade or your problem is still as upsetting as when you began, make sure you are following the Five Simple Steps. Perhaps you are leaving out the affirmation or skipping one or more energy points. Reread Chapter 2 carefully and follow the instructions as described.

Many people report that saying the affirmation dramatically with a forceful voice while tapping the Karate Chop spot or rubbing the Tender spot on the upper chest increases the effectiveness of the process. Say the affirmation with feeling and notice what happens. Yell it out in a loud voice. Tap the Karate Chop point or rub the Tender spot more often.

That's Not the Issue

In step one of the Five Simple Steps you choose the problem or negative emotion you want to neutralize. At times, Meridian Therapy won't seem to work because you are focusing on the wrong problem. The real problem may be hiding behind the problem you are trying to treat. Emma tried to work on her fear of flying and got poor results. The more she tapped, the more frustrated she became because her fear didn't diminish.

She discovered that the main problem was not her fear of flying, but rather her need to always be in a state of worry. According to Emma, "Someone's got to worry. That's how it's always been in my family. My husband won't worry, so I have to." Emma's negative core belief was, "If I give up my worry about flying something terrible will happen to me or my loved ones." When she dealt with her belief about the importance of worry as her main problem, she found that flying became less stressful.

Biting Off Too Much

You may be tapping daily about a long-standing problem and notice that only minor changes are taking place. It doesn't mean that Meridian Therapy isn't working. Progress is slower when you tap about broad topics. When you say, "Even though I have this eating disorder or general anxiety, trauma, insomnia, or procrastination," you are treating it very broadly. These conditions are complex. Within each one are many negative emotions such as fear, anxiety, guilt, shame, anger, and sadness. Many memories that span years of your life can influence a long-standing issue.

Break the problem down into specific parts, moments, or events. When Gwen started tapping about her eating disorder, she felt only a little better and didn't notice much change in her binge behavior. After she named "sugar craving" as one of the components of her problem, she saw a change immediately. When she tapped about eating "too large portions," it brought up her fear of deprivation. Tapping about each of the things she felt powerless over in her life helped her become aware of the situations that triggered her cravings. As a result, she began to notice significant changes in her compulsive behavior and had fewer binges.

You will have more success dealing with insomnia if you delineate the way you experience the problem. Do you have trouble falling asleep, staying asleep, waking early, or a combination of these? When did the problem start? What are the characteristics of the problem: wide awake at 4:00 A.M., tossing and turning for an hour at bedtime, nightmares' waking you up, waking an hour before your alarm, lying awake with racing thoughts? By tapping on the specific characteristics of your problem, you will see faster results.

In the chapters that deal with compulsion, panic, trauma, and procrastination, I guide you to look for special memories, relationships, habits, and beliefs. As you use Meridian Therapy for each one, you reduce the size of the overall problem more rapidly than if you treat the problem globally. Seek professional help to guide you through complicated problems if you are feeling bogged down.

Dealing with Aspects

When you seem to be skipping around to new memories, thoughts, or feelings with each round of tapping, it doesn't mean you are doing it incorrectly or that Meridian Therapy isn't working. You are experiencing *aspects*. Aspects are the facets of the problem. Each round of tapping is like peeling an onion. As one thought or feeling is relieved, it makes room for another to surface. That's what happened to Chloe.

As a part-time college student, Chloe had very little money and was between jobs. She was depressed when she called me. I arranged to work with her at a special student rate. She wanted to focus on raising her self-esteem. During one session we were working on a problem about her family when, after a round of tapping, I asked her if she noticed anything. Chloe appeared flustered and said, "I guess I'm not doing this right. My mind was wandering." Often, when an aspect appears, people think their mind is wandering because they seem to have strayed from the original topic. I asked Chloe what her wandering thoughts were. She said, "I was thinking about how you see me for so little money and wondered why someone like you would do that for a person like me." She was not doing Meridian Therapy wrong, rather she was continuing to uncover facets of her problem. Her thoughts were revealing how her low self-regard affected all her relationships. *I don't deserve* was one of her most insidious blocking beliefs.

A Path in the Forest

Problems are like trees. Some are tall and some short. Some are large with enormous thick trunks and others are mere saplings. There are times in our lives when we feel lost in the forest and can't seem to find our way out. As you use Meridian Therapy you will be able to cut down the trees that are barring your path.

Small trees represent problems that are easy to tap away. Larger trees have many roots and branches. If you think of a tree trunk as representing the major problem or emotion you are working to heal, branches are variations of the same topic. Not all problems are so simple that the negative charge dissipates in two or three rounds. Newcomers to Meridian Therapy sometimes believe they aren't doing it right because as they tap the energy points, new thoughts, feelings, or memories pop up that seem to lead them away from the original problem.

Following the Branches

When one thing leads to another and another, I call them "branches." Julio, a forty-five-year-old teacher, was suffering from post-traumatic stress symptoms after an auto accident in which he was shaken up but not severely injured. He began with an anxiety level at nine. As he tapped he remembered moments from the accident, the noise of impact and hitting his head. Next he recalled having the wind knocked out of him. Then he remembered another car accident he had many years ago. After that he recalled still another fender bender. It took only two more rounds of tapping until his discomfort about the previous accidents was neutralized.

Branches consist of new material that is related to the starting issue or has some similarity to it. Julio's tapping brought up a series of similar memories of other accidents that affected his present distress. As he tapped, his emotions changed. Each new feeling or topic is like a new branch that has its own twigs attached. It is important to follow whatever arises and trust that each piece is a part of the whole tree and needs to be healed.

Julio remembered a variety of accidents when he tried to heal a recent one. Fifty-year-old Reva thought of different codependent relationships she had previously engaged in, while working on the loss of her twenty-year marriage to an alcoholic. Remembering a series of like events while tapping is a common experience.

Reva was using Meridian Therapy to relieve loneliness and unhappiness about her inability to find romance after her divorce. At first tapping brought up branches as she remembered some of her other relationships with men she had tried to "rescue," just like her ex-husband. Her belief that everyone let her down created another branch.

Stumbling Over the Roots

Then Reva stumbled over a "root," an underlying core issue that feeds the current problem just as the root of the tree, buried below the surface, feeds it. Reva realized that among those who let her down was her mother. A few more rounds of tapping brought up great anger toward her mother for neglecting Reva when her sister was born. Reva felt despair as she thought about that time. She said, "Even though I was such a good girl it didn't help. She never paid attention to my needs." As Reva recollected the memories about her codependent relationships and her unhappy childhood, she realized that early in life she had decided that she would never get what she wanted, no matter how good she was. She kept picking men who didn't or couldn't give her what she never got and desperately wanted from her mother. This root was deep below the surface of her conscious mind.

Roots are thoughts, feelings, or memories about other areas of your life that do not immediately seem to relate to what you are focusing on but are at the heart of the problem. Reva switched from thinking about romantic relationships to remembering how her mother acted when her sister was born. Strong emotions about her mother and decisions she made about who she was and what kind of life she deserved affected her adult love relationships. Although a root may seem like an entirely new topic, it is related.

When the Upset Remains

When beginning the Five Simple Steps, it is important to ask yourself to rate the negative charge or emotion you are feeling. If, after going through the procedure a few times, your level of distress remains the same, you may have hit a root or some branches. Notice any new thoughts or sensations and tap about them. If the intensity of the negative feeling eases somewhat and then grows strong again, perhaps you addressed the problem too generally. Break it down into smaller segments. This is especially true for physical pain. When pain returns it can be a manifestation of an emotional issue that needs to be treated.

Another hint: When the level of upset doesn't budge, observe where in your body you feel the negative charge most strongly. Then try one or more of these suggestions:

- Focus on the body feeling without words and tap a few rounds. The sensation may travel to another part of the body. Just follow it until there is no negative charge and the body feels relaxed.
- Think about what the disturbance in the body looks like. Does it have a color, texture, size, or shape? Bring this to mind as you feel it strongly within. Then tap.
- Is there a word that goes with the feeling inside? Think of that word and tap.

Polarity Switching

Sometimes psychological and physical problems are slow to respond because there is a disruption in the body's energy system. Kinesiologists refer to this as "switching." Others call it "neurological disorganization." The body has a north and south pole the same as a battery. Reversal of the poles can result from structural imbalance in the body, exposure to foods or substances you are sensitive to, or psychological stress. People whose energy is switched often have difficulties with physical coordination. If this is a chronic problem you may want to seek treatment from a chiropractor, osteopath, or cranio-sacral specialist.

Cook's Hook-Up

Wayne Cook, an expert on electromagnetic energy, created a simple exercise to stimulate energy and balance the brain. It is usually referred to as "Cook's Hook-Up." You can do this seated or standing up.

- Clasp your hands together and notice whether the right or left thumb is on top.
- Unclasp hands. Extend your arms in front of you with the backs of the hands facing each other and the palms facing out.
- Take the hand that had the thumb on top and raise it up and over the other hand so they are palm to palm. Now intertwine the fingers of both hands together.
- Bend your elbows and bring your entwined hands down, under and against your chest.
- If your right thumb was on top, cross the right ankle over the left. If your left thumb was on top, cross your left ankle over the right ankle.
- Touch the tip of your tongue to the roof of your mouth behind the front teeth.
- Close your eyes, breathing naturally. If you are standing keep your eyes open. Hold this for thirty seconds.
- Uncross your legs.

- Place the fingertips of both hands together to form a teepee. Keep your eyes closed, tongue touching roof of mouth, breathing naturally. Hold this for thirty to sixty seconds.

Energy Toxins

There may also be physical problems that interfere with the Meridian Therapy outcome. After treating herself with Meridian Therapy for anxiety, Gayle, who suffered from extreme panic attacks, was excited when her panic attacks began to disappear. On a beautiful Saturday, when she was looking forward to a happy family day, panic suddenly took over. Panic attacks upset her for most of the day. Meridian Therapy did not help. Afterward she remembered that she had drunk coffee that morning. The caffeine upset her body and triggered panic. For Gayle caffeine is an *energy toxin*. After she refrained from drinking coffee, the experience of nonstop panic was gone for good.

Energy toxins are substances that disturb the body's energy. Many people who are sensitive to such things as wheat, corn, sugar, and food additives feel physically uncomfortable and may also be affected emotionally. Caffeine and alcohol can be toxic, as can substances we apply to our bodies such as deodorant, hair spray, cosmetics, or laundry detergent. Particles in the air you breathe may have a negative effect. If you are abusing drugs, you may also experience this problem.

When you are able to reduce your level of emotional discomfort to zero, but the negative emotion keeps coming back, this is another indication that energy toxins are the problem. You may have exposed yourself to a food or substance a few hours before using the tapping technique, and you are feeling the adverse results.

Test Yourself for Allergens

In his book *The Pulse Test*, Arthur Coca, M.D., uses the pulse as a guide to good health. Dr. Coca believes that allergens speed up the pulse. He outlines a simple system for testing yourself for allergens. Part of his plan consists of taking your pulse upon awakening, again just before eating a single food, then a half-hour after eating, and finally an hour after eating. If the pulse rate exceeds your normal pulse rate, you may be sensitive to the food. As you eliminate the foods that raise your pulse rate, you will feel better and respond more positively to Meridian Therapy. If you know that you are sensitive to substances you ingest or breathe, consult someone who specializes in treating this type of problem.

You're on Your Way!

You now know how to do Meridian Therapy in Five Simple Steps and variations of the Five Simple Steps. You have ideas and instructions for applying Meridian Therapy to free you from many kinds of psychological problems, negative emotions, and pain. When you make Meridian Therapy part of your daily life, you will experience less depression and more joy. Problem-solving will become easier as you tap your way beyond anxiety and fear.

Your Pet's Best Friend: How to Treat Animals with Meridian Therapy

Many of us feel closely bonded to our pets. We love them, and they return that love. Pets seem especially attuned to the energy of certain people. One of our cats knows when my husband is nearing home and waits at the door before he approaches the driveway. In his book *Dogs That Know When Their Owners Are Coming Home*, Dr. Rupert Sheldrake attempts to explain this phenomenon and other amazing animal behavior. Two thousand pet owners, animal trainers, handlers, breeders, and veterinarians helped Dr. Sheldrake during five years of extensive research.

Sheldrake believes that pet owners telepathically communicate their intention to come home. Many pets get excited and display a special behavior at the moment when the owner is leaving a faroff place and heading home. There are even cats and dogs that know when their owner is the one on the other end of the line when the telephone rings. Some pets respond to the silent call of their owner and others react when their owner is in distress or dying far away.

A Special Connection

Dr. Sheldrake maintains that humans and their pets are connected within Morphic fields that link all the members of a social group. People and their animal companions might be considered a group. The Morphic field embraces all these members within itself. A member who goes any distance away from the group still remains connected through this field because Morphic fields seem able to stretch like invisible rubber bands. Therefore, it is possible for them to act as channels for telepathic communication even over enormous distances. This finding comes as no surprise to many of us animal lovers.

Because of the bond between people and their pets, it is possible to treat animals with Meridian Therapy or use surrogate tapping. Pet owners can tap themselves in place of the upset animal while thinking about their pet's problem. Here are some stories about animal lovers and their pets that I have collected from pet lovers.

Helping Junior to Pee

My cat Junior is eleven and has a problem common among male cats. His plumbing gets blocked every so often and he can't pee. This is either stress- or food-induced and flares up about once a year or so, requiring an expensive trip to the vet.

All day Friday I noticed he would go in the litterbox and sit and wait and nothing would come out, a sure sign the plumbing was blocked again. He was clearly in stress and pain. I put Junior on a piece of carpet in the garage and did a round of surrogate tapping saying, "Even though I can't pee . . ." After one round, Junior stood up and walked off the carpet, leaving a huge puddle behind him. I was blown away. I kept close watch on him during the night and he was completely fine and back to normal.

Michelle L.

No More Wrestling

I've been a "doubting Thomas" about the idea that intention will work with animals. However, I experimented in spite of the doubts and have had some fairly solid results on two of my three dogs. We took my biggest Newfoundland to the vet with a bad ear infection in the left ear. She needs to have special cream in her ear daily. She does not want anyone to touch it. In fact, for two days she won wrestling matches when I tried to hold her down while my wife put the medicine in her ear. I tried surrogate tapping for her resistance. The change is like night and day. For three days there has been no more wrestling. She still doesn't like it and occasionally shakes her head when the medicine is about to go in, but it's definitely doable.

We've been having sewer and water main pipes put in the roads near our house this past week. This has really upset the oldest and smallest of our cocker spaniels. She barked constantly while they worked, and I do mean constantly, enough to make even me upset with her. I did the surrogate animal tapping, and it reduced the problem 80 to 90 percent.

Tom K.

Afraid of Thunder

I am amazed at the change in our family's shivering, teeth-chattering, drooling-in-a-thunderstorm dog after my wife and I began surrogate tapping for this poor critter's obvious symptoms of distress. There were selfish motives on our part, since the dog stood over our pillow in the middle of the night to exhibit this behavior. There was no sleep in our house unless one of us got up and moved to the couch in the other room with the dog, so the one remaining in bed could sleep.

Years ago we went on a vacation and boarded the dog at the vet. We returned to find a raw spot on her leg where she'd been licking. The spot never went away. She kept it open with licking. Since we've surrogate-tapped for "calm feelings" during the thunderstorms, the spot is drying up. There is still no hair and there is a big raised, callus-looking thing on the leg, but there is no seepage. And she's stopped licking it at all.

Tom B.

A Scaredy-Cat Dog

My neighbor Beth has a dog she rescued from the pound, Yellow, who is frightened of just about everything, most noticeably other dogs, cats, and Beth's wood floors. Yellow had slowly become a little less nervous about life over the last two years or so. Recently when Yellow was in Beth's car by himself there was an explosion nearby, which broke Beth's car window, and Yellow completely regressed. He became afraid to leave Beth's side.

Beth, the cat, and I sat on the couch, and Yellow was in a

chair across the room. We did several rounds of tapping over the course of half an hour. Beth thought about various incidents and situations in which she has observed Yellow being frightened. She tapped on herself for each of them.

Afterward, I went home and got my dog, a beautifully exuberant one-and-a-half-year-old that has always intimidated Yellow with her playfulness. For the first time, Yellow stayed in the yard with Beth, me, and my dog. Later, Yellow played in the house, another first, and ran across the wood floors without a thought. Before the tapping treatment Yellow would not walk on the wood floors. Yellow is a happier, more sociable dog since Meridian Therapy changed his life.

Mary S.

I Won't Go!

Yesterday I had to take my cat to the vet for annual shots. That's not the problem—getting her into the carrying cage is! I was looking at her at breakfast time and tapping on myself affirming that she was a wonderful cat in spite of her reluctance to get in the cage to transport her to the office. No problem. She sat docilely on the examining table and even cuddled up to the vet.

Maureen M.

Help Me Make It Through the Night

We have taken in a rescued wolfhound and for the first few days he was obviously finding his feet and getting used to us and our home. The night before last he was unhappy about being locked up for the night. I'd hardly gotten into bed before he started banging at the door and whining, barking, and howling. I got very little sleep and eventually gave up at 5:00 A.M. and took him out.

Last night the same thing started but this time, probably through desperation, I started tapping about his anxiety and distress. I'd hardly gotten half way through the first round when he was quiet, but I completed the round and did a round on his insecurity. Then I finished off with one suggesting that he could sleep comfortably through the night. I don't know whether he actually did that, of course, but he was quiet all night. I've since tapped again on his insecurity and he is much calmer and sleeping more.

Hilary J.

A Dog Sitter's Report

Hi Sandy,

Well, I just want to tell you how it went today. Woody is not easy. When I arrived he was barking to go out as usual. I mean nonstop. I tried to get him to sit for a moment and that was unsuccessful, so I proceeded to rub on the Tender spot and said, "Although Woody has anxiety he will stop his barking." After a few moments I once again told him to sit and be patient. He did. He sat and looked up at me. We made good eye contact as I continued to tap myself for him. He actually sat quietly for a few minutes while I got his collar to take him for his walk.

We had a good walk. When we return he usually begins his barking again, but he didn't. He sat quietly while I got him a cookie. This was very good because Woody barks a lot. I will see him again later and will do more tapping to try to relax him. Feel free to pass this on to others. Talk with you later.

Ginny the Pet Sitter
Sandra H.

Sophie's Arthritis

My fourteen-year-old golden retriever Sophie has had arthritis since she was six.We've helped her with nutrition, herbs, homoeopathy, and acupuncture, but it stays in the background. Last week her front right paw swelled up so much that it became deformed. I tapped on myself for her, affirming, "Even though Sophie has a painful swollen paw . . ." and "Even though Sophie has arthritis . . ." I couldn't believe my eyes. The swelling went down as though it were a balloon letting out air. It was like a horror story special effect in reverse.

I didn't trust myself not to have imagined it, but Sophie was good enough to manifest the swollen paw while my sister was visiting. I again tapped while she and my husband looked on. Again, we saw the swelling subside in front of our eyes. You couldn't have more positive proof that surrogate tapping works. My sister hurried home to tap on her own dogs.

Catherine D.

Death of a Pet

This morning, I went upstairs on a hunch and found our old dog Charlie dead in my bedroom. Only minutes before she had run around the garden, barking at birds. My young son, age nine, insisted I take her to the vet to make her better and got quite hysterical. I tapped to calm him and then could explain how it was an amazing death, without pain or suffering, and that she was waiting in the light until we came along one day.

My eighteen-year-old son couldn't go upstairs. He's had a phobia to do with dead things since he turned eight. He knows how to treat himself with Meridian Therapy and thought it was a good day to let this fear finally go. He tapped himself from one step to the next, and eventually, with my support, made it into the bedroom to be able to say goodbye to Charlie.

We then all took her body to be cremated, and when I got home, I sat in a corner and tapped myself for my great sadness, because one bereavement tends to link into all bereavements, until I felt calm and grateful for Charlie's great gifts of friendliness, happiness, and positivity. What a wonderful thing it is to be able to help one's children in such a concrete way.

Silvia K.

Suggested Reading

Arenson, Gloria. *How to Stop Playing the Weighting Game*. New York: St. Martin's Press, 1981.

————. *A Substance Called Food: How to Understand, Control and Recover from Addictive Eating*. Pennsylvania: Tab Books, 1989.

————. *Conquering Compulsive Behavior* (audiocassette). Los Angeles: 1989.

————. *Born to Spend*. Pennsylvania: Tab Books, 1991.

Beck, Aaron T. *Cognitive Therapy and the Emotional Disorders*. New York: Meridian, 1976.

Becker, Robert O. *The Body Electric*. New York: William Morrow, 1985.

Burns, David D. *Feeling Good: The New Mood Therapy*. New York: Morrow, 1980.

Burr, Harold S. *Blueprint for Immortality: The Electric Patterns of Life*. Essex, England: Neville Spearman Publishers, 1972.

Callahan, R. J. *Five Minute Phobia Cure*. Wilmington, Del.: Enterprise, 1985.

Callahan, R. J., and Callahan, J. *Thought Field Therapy and Trauma: Treatment and Theory*. Indian Wells, Calif.: Self-Published, 1996.

Craig, Gary. *Steps toward Becoming the Ultimate Therapist* (video) Sea Ranch, Calif.: 1998.

Craig, Gary, and Fowlie, Adrienne. *Emotional Freedom Techniques* (video). Sea Ranch, Calif.: 1995.

Diamond, John. *Your Body Doesn't Lie*. New York: Warner Books, 1979.

Durlacher, James V. *Freedom from Fear Forever*. Tempe, Ariz.: Van Ness Publishing Co., 1994.

Eden, Donna, and Feinstein, David. *Energy Medicine: Balance Your Body's Energies for Optimum Health, Joy and Vitality.* New York: Jeremy Tarcher/Putnam, 1999.

Gallo, Fred. *Energy Psychology: Explorations at the Interface of Energy, Cognition, Behavior, and Health.* Boca Raton, Fla.:CRC Press, 1999.

Gerber, Richard. *Vibrational Medicine.* Santa Fe, N.Mex.: Bear & Co, 1996.

Jacobs, Gregg D. *Say Goodnight to Insomnia.* New York: Henry Holt & Co., 1998.

Lambrou, Peter, and Pratt, George G. *Instant Emotional Healing: Acupressure for the Emotions.* New York: Broadway Books, 2000.

Milkman, Harvey, and Sunderwirth, Stanley. *Craving for Ecstasy.* Lexington, Mass.: Lexington Books, 1987.

Myss, Caroline. *Anatomy of the Spirit.* New York: Harmony Books, 1996.

Pert, Candace B. *Molecules of Emotion.* New York: Scribner's. 1997.

Rubik, Beverly. *Life at the Edge of Science.* Philadelphia: Institute for Frontier Science, 1996.

Ruden, Ronald. *The Craving Brain.* New York: Harper Collins, 1997.

Sheldrake, Rupert. *Dogs That Know When Their Owners Are Coming Home.* New York: Crown Publishers, 1999.

Teplitz, Jerry V. and Eckroate, Norma. *Switched-On Living.* Norfolk, Va.: Hampton Roads, 1994.

Tiller, W. A. *Science and Human Transformation: Subtle Energies, Intentionality and Consciousness.* California: Pavior, 1997.

Resources

Association for Comprehensive Energy Psychology
www.energypsych.org
International organization for the practice of energy psychology

Be Set Free Fast
Larry Phillip Nims, Ph.D.
www.besetfreefast.com

Emotional Freedom Techniques ™
Gary H. Craig
www.emofree.com

Energy Diagnostic and Treatment Methods (EDx™)
Fred Gallo, Ph.D.
www.energypsych.com

Meridian Therapy
Gloria Arenson, MS, MFT
www.meridianpsychotherapy.com

Thought Energy Synchronization Therapies (TEST)
Greg Nicosia, Ph.D.
www.thoughtenergy.com

Thought Field Therapy
Callahan Techniques, Ltd.
www.tftrx.com

Index